THE THIRTEENTH STEP

MARKUS HEILIG

THE THIRTEENTH STEP

Addiction in the Age of Brain Science

Columbia University Press / New York

Columbia University Press
Publishers Since 1893
New York   Chichester, West Sussex
cup.columbia.edu
Copyright © 2015 Markus Heilig

Library of Congress Cataloging-in-Publication Data

Heilig, Markus, author.
   The thirteenth step : addiction in the age of brain science / Markus Heilig.
      p. ; cm.
   Includes bibliographical references and index.
   ISBN 978-0-231-17236-3 (cloth : alk. paper) — ISBN 978-0-231-53902-9 (e-book)
   I. Title.
   [DNLM: 1. Substance-Related Disorders—therapy.   2. Alcoholism—therapy.
3. Behavior, Addictive—metabolism.   4. Brain—drug effects.   5. Brain—physiopa-
thology.   6. Pharmacogenetics.   WM 270]

RC564
616.86'061—dc23   2014022405

COVER DESIGN: *Noah Arlow*

References to websites (URLs) were accurate at the time of writing. Neither the author
nor Columbia University Press is responsible for URLs that may have expired or
changed since the manuscript was prepared.

CONTENTS

CONTENTS

ACKNOWLEDGMENTS

I am indebted to more people than I can list—family, friends, colleagues, collaborators, coworkers, competitors, and patients. Some deserve special thanks:

Claes Wahlestedt has been a friend and collaborator for some twenty-five years. As a fellow research student, he pulled me into the fascinating world of neuropharmacology, and he has since always enriched my thinking with his exciting perspective, often very different from my own yet so complementary.

Erik Widerlöv was many years ago my thesis adviser and was able to strike the perfect balance between guidance and freedom, allowing me to grow in the early stages of my training as a physician and research student.

Jörgen Engel introduced me to the neuroscience of addiction; Bob Murison helped me as I moved into behavioral pharmacology. Both have remained dear friends.

George Koob, currently the director of the National Institute on Alcohol Abuse and Alcoholism in Bethesda, Maryland, was once my postdoctoral mentor at the Scripps Research Institute in La Jolla, California. That experience continued to inspire me for many years.

Marie Åsberg supported me when I was starting my own research program and became a role model. A lunch with Marie remains the most reliable cure for a temporary loss of inspiration.

Lars Gunne, one of the pioneers of methadone maintenance treatment, taught me to combine scientific rigor with empathy and respect for patients with addictive disorders, in a field where those elements are too often lacking.

Rainer Spanagel, Roberto Ciccocioppo, and Donald Gehlert are remarkable scientists and great friends whom I too rarely get to see or collaborate with these days.

Daniel Hommer was a wonderful physician scientist, a close collaborator who taught me much of what I know about brain imaging, and a friend whose generosity and big heart touched us all. Tragically, Dan died while this book was being written, leaving a huge void in our lives.

Yavin Shaham and his wife, Karin Helmers, are the best friends anyone could ever wish for. Yavin is a stellar neuroscientist, a true scholar, and a model of integrity and generosity. Without his friendship, I don't know how I would have gotten through some difficult times. Without his scholarship, I would not know half of what I know.

I am indebted to countless patients encountered over some twenty-five years. Many have taken journeys that were painful to follow, but sharing their experience has also frequently been heartwarming and enlightening. Occasionally sharing the joy of life winning out over disease is the ultimate award in my line of work.

Numerous people at the Hazelden Foundation, Center City, Minnesota, were immensely helpful as I was developing this project. I am particularly grateful to President and CEO Mark Mishek; Provost Valery Slaymaker of the Hazelden Graduate School of Addiction Studies; and Professionals in Residence Program Specialist Roxanne McGurk.

Many members of my research group, past and present, have become a second family and enabled me to do most of what I have done. Over time and on both sides of the Atlantic, we have learned together, developed concepts, generated data, shared joys and sorrows, and had fun while trying to remember why we do what we do—because patients need it. As is the nature of this strange, nomadic science life, people have moved to other countries, other fields, their own labs, or clinical work. I proudly follow the careers of former trainees as they build their own research groups or clinical programs. They include Roberto Rimondini at Bologna University, Italy;

Annika Thorsell at Linköping University, Sweden; Wolfgang Sommer and Anita Hansson in Mannheim, Germany; Christina Barr at the National Institute on Alcohol Abuse and Alcoholism; Åsa Magnusson at the Karolinska Institute; and Jesse Schank at University of Georgia, to name a few. Among the current crew, staff scientists Jenica Tapocik and Melanie Schwandt are as appreciated as they are indispensible. As for the postdocs still in the lab, get a job and I'll name you in the next edition!

Helena, Sara, and Hanna, my three muses, and Johan and Martin, my guy friends in the family, have given meaning to it all and made my work possible by following me wherever it has taken me. They have also provided all the distraction from science I will ever need. Their happiness means more to me than anything else.

This book is dedicated to the memory of my father. One of the toughest men I have ever met, he once turned himself in to the Gestapo in exchange for his little brother, only to live seven decades past the death sentence brought upon him by that action. Rising from the ashes of the Holocaust, he devoted his life to my mother, me, and my sister. To create opportunities for us, he left behind a successful career and a home in Poland and started over in Sweden in 1970. He always expected as much of himself as he did of others; from my earliest years, it was clear that nothing short of solid work would win his approval. Yet he was always there in an hour of need and never stopped looking out for us, even in the end, when he was the one in need of support. The best I can hope for is to be half as good a father as he was.

THE THIRTEENTH STEP

1

US AND THEM

A S THE NURSE on the floor picked up the chart to read the transfer note, she thought there must have been a mix-up. She sighed. It was a Friday afternoon, and, like her colleagues, she was getting ready to get off her shift and go home. She was a good nurse, one of many in the underappreciated army who keep hospitals going by juggling a job and family. On any other day, she did not mind unexpected work. In fact she enjoyed it, thriving on getting things right, offering comfort to patients, and keeping physicians in line. After fifteen years in the profession, much of it had become routine. For the most part that was a good thing, relieving her of the anxieties of the early years and allowing her to spend more time with patients, the most gratifying part of the job. But this once she was not really into it. She had expected to reclaim some hard-earned comp time and for once leave early so she could get to the grocery store before it was invaded by hordes of other suburbanites. Instead here it was: a last-minute transfer from the medical floor in anticipation of a busy weekend.

In the rush, something seemed to have become mixed up. The label on the chart identified the patient as a fifty-two-year-old woman. Instead the patient in front of the nurse looked like she was closer to eighty and dying. Yellow as a canary, she looked shrunken and could not have weighed over eighty pounds, yet her belly floated out into the bed like a balloon half filled with water. Her body was covered with sores and bruises, making her look like she had been badly beaten. To an experienced eye, however, it was one of the unmistakable signs of advanced liver failure—when platelet counts are so low they cannot plug little holes in broken blood vessels, and coagulation factors that could start the repair process are also largely absent because the liver cannot make enough of them. The nurse greeted the patient and tried to get the usual admission talk going, but after a polite initial response, the patient excused herself, saying that she felt terribly tired, and asked the nurse to please read the chart for her history so she could rest. She then turned toward the wall and became quiet, maybe falling back into a shallow sleep, maybe just resting. As she breathed, a sickeningly sweet smell filled the room.

The chart offered an equally conflicting story. The patient was a married homemaker who lived in a single-family home in a well-to-do suburb, not too far from where the nurse herself lived. Two children, both boys, now studying at the city's prestigious Institute of Technology and living in the college dorms, were mentioned. The history of prior contacts with the health care system was very limited. There was reference to some old prescriptions for insomnia from the family doctor. There was mention of a round of referrals over the past couple of years to evaluate possible causes of an accelerating weight loss. A routine workup to rule out cancer showed no significant findings. And then there were a couple of admissions for abdominal pain, which were written off as the result of emotional distress caused by the departure of the grown children.

But just over two weeks ago, the patient's husband had found her unconscious when he returned from a business trip. She was brought to the emergency room, and the admission exam showed life-threatening liver failure. Her urine output had rapidly decreased and there was fluid in her abdomen and blood in her stools. An ultrasound of the liver had shown an organ that was shrunk and nodular, like a cluster of grapes, rather than the normal healthy smoothness. Only the miracles of modern medicine, including a stint in the intensive care unit, had kept her alive. After the ICU she had been stabilized on the medical floor, with continued intravenous fluids, platelet transfusions, and fresh frozen plasma. Yet for all the advances of medicine, and all the scientifically derived algorithms that spit out prognostic numbers, no one knew whether she would make it. It seemed from the progress notes that both staff and family had written her off. Her sons had been contacted, came to visit in disbelief, and left hours later with ashen faces, to return a couple more times before they dropped off the radar screen. Her husband, though, had stayed night after night until things seemed to slowly start turning around, and he returned daily during visiting hours, a quiet shadow.

It was only in the transfer note from the medical unit that heavy use of alcohol was mentioned, for the first time, as the reason this otherwise healthy, affluent mother of two had been so close to dying of liver failure.

The nurse closed the chart, quietly shaking her head in disbelief. She worked in a psychiatric addiction unit. The doctors and nurses prided themselves on being unfazed by almost any human behavior or predicament. The drugs, the addictions, the withdrawals were just the beginning, and staff had the routines for managing those down to the tiniest detail. And they had pretty much seen it all. One patient could be an unruly 250-pound port worker who had gone into a classic delirium tremens after having been admitted for chest pain and having his alcohol supply cut off. Another could be an old lady with quiet delusions signifying the onset of a late delirium from Valium overuse. Or perhaps, hiding under the use of tranquilizers, a true delusional syndrome lurked, the vast labyrinths of which suddenly opened in response to a single trigger word, which unleashed paranoid stories. The staff were acutely aware that seemingly strange behavior could occasionally be the result of or mask a serious medical condition. While trying to help and comfort people, they had to make sure no drugs entered the unit and that no medical condition was missed. In short, the psychiatric addiction unit was a challenging but fascinating place to work.

Whether a patient came in from the emergency room or from another unit in the hospital, or was a scheduled admission from the outside, there was a strict admission policy. It included thoroughly searching anything that was brought into the unit and strip searching the patient. Newcomers on staff sometimes rebelled against this. They brought up patients' rights, autonomy, and respect. The most experienced nurses sighed and then tried to explain. A few of the new staff never got it and moved on to other units. The vast majority noticed that patients had no problem with the routines if they were done right and quickly absorbed the healthy "tough love" culture of the unit. Like their more seasoned colleagues, most newcomers ultimately learned to set boundaries with care, making it clear that allowing patients opportunities to overdose in the hospital or sell drugs to other patients was impermissible.

But this case was different. The prematurely aged woman lay there, turned away from the nurse in the still and peaceful room. It was as if death had entered the hospital and then decided it was not yet time to claim the patient. It felt out of place—in fact, inappropriate—to disturb the patient and start searching her and her belongings. The nurse sighed again, completed the transfer sheet, and started rolling the bed from the admission room onto the unit, with the patient's neatly packed bag underneath it. As she was rolling the bed down the corridor, she saw the young psychiatry resident who would have to complete the admission. She waved, pointed to the room where the patient was going to be placed, and moved on. Poor guy, she thought. He would have to stay even longer than she did. Then she reconsidered. After all, he didn't have any kids to feed tonight. And besides, those guys all went on to make twice the money she did, or more. There was really no reason to pity him. She pushed the bed to the wall, secured the wheels, and quietly left the ward for the world outside.

By Monday morning the patient was dead. Hidden in her bag had been a quart of vodka. She had consumed almost all of it before anyone had noticed. After that she had become unconscious and, despite efforts to revive her, died within a few hours.

Addictive disorders kill and debilitate countless people, most of whom are in the prime of their lives. Alcohol alone ranks as the third most common preventable cause of death in the United States and is estimated by the Centers for Disease Control and Prevention (CDC) to kill an astounding eighty to ninety thousand people each year.[1] On average, the lives of these people are shortened by about thirty years. Among preventable causes of death, alcohol is topped only by smoking and a lifestyle of physical inactivity and unhealthy diet. In an increasingly health-conscious society, not a week goes by without reminders of public health and personal consequences caused by such factors. The pharmaceutical industry invests billions of dollars in developing antismoking as well as antiobesity drugs. In contrast, rarely does alcohol or other drug addiction receive similar attention. When it does, it is often in the guise of other issues. Car crashes and other accidents cause about forty thousand alcohol-related deaths. Liver cirrhosis, cancer, and other medical conditions caused by excessive alcohol use result in thirty-five thousand more. Frequently those conditions receive more attention and sympathy than the underlying addiction. It is a bit like being concerned that patients die because their heart stops beating but neglecting to consider the hypertension that caused that to happen. Beyond the deaths, the CDC has estimated the annual economic cost of damage inflicted by alcohol and other drugs as over a quarter trillion dollars in the United States alone. No numbers, however, can properly capture the emotional toll of addictive disorders.

All too often people have little sympathy for the plight of alcohol or drug addicts. "It is self-inflicted." "They should just get their act together." "Just say no." "Lock them up." This phenomenon is as interesting as it is disturbing. Don't people generally hold that if you have a home, an income, a family, and perhaps even a sense of meaning to your life, then you are obliged to give some thought to those less fortunate than yourself? Yet people persist in a lack of compassion for those suffering from addictive disorders. What allows for this apparent contradiction to continue is a split that is as basic as it is false. Even otherwise caring people routinely make a distinction between "us," the good citizens who deserve a helping hand when we fall on hard times, and "them," the fundamentally different people on the margin who may smell bad, stagger, scream, behave in bizarre ways in the metro, or stop breathing on the floor of a public restroom.

If you, too, hold this belief, I have a surprise for you. Your brain is not wired much differently from that of your fellow human on that floor. Understanding the neurobiology of addictive behavior, if only to the degree possible at present, is a good vaccine against drawing lines between "us" and "them." Drugs hook into brain circuitry we all rely on to obtain what we desire, avoid dangers, and make sensible decisions. Once you have realized that, it is impossible to look at a person with an addiction and escape the thought, "There, but for the grace of God, go I."

Had it not been for some unexpected turns of life, I might never have learned these lessons. Born into the protected environment of an academic family, I had as a child only once seen anyone intoxicated, when a colonel in the Polish Army got down on the floor during a dinner party my parents hosted, held his pistol in his teeth by the trigger guard, and ran around barking like a dog. But at the age of eleven, I was thrown into a world I had until then not known existed. Our family became refugees from the latest persecutions of Polish Jews and ended up in a small town in the south of Sweden, by way of first an Italian and then a Swedish refugee camp. We left behind virtually all we had owned and settled down in an area to which others who owned little or nothing also gravitated. Drugs and violence were commonplace. In memory, this period of my life lies between two land-marks. The first was an early bike trip to the grocery store for my mother, interrupted by a knife threat from a guy who, I now realize, must have been high on amphetamine. The second was an encounter, many years later, at an outdoor café across the street from the eleventh-century Romanesque cathedral that towers over the city of my alma mater. My parents and I were quietly celebrating my graduation from medical school at the oldest coffee shop in town, now gone. I can still see my former classmate from grade school, Ante, crossing the street and heading toward us, smiling, waving his hand, happy to see me, but already visibly intoxicated at the noon hour. He quickly dismissed our unspoken reaction. He was just out of jail, he told us, did not expect to stay on the outside long, and intended to make the best of the time available to him. In between those two memory landmarks, kids I knew succumbed to drugs. One died from a heroin overdose. Another was killed when he drove his motorcycle while intoxicated and was hit by a truck.

I have since spent more than twenty years working with psychiatric and addictive disorders. As a young physician I had patients who made it and those who did not. I was vomited on, given flowers, lied to, told heart-wrenching life stories, threatened, or hugged, in a kaleidoscopic stream of experience. I felt hopeful at times but powerless much more often. I saw how the medical model, helpful though I found it, was also painfully insufficient in dealing with addictions. Recognizing the limitations of a hospital, my colleagues and I worked hard to establish mobile services and reach out to those whose addiction had made them homeless, whose homelessness had made them addicted, or for whom one simply could not tease out what might have caused what. As "treatment" we would listen, talk, and give behavioral therapies and medicines, but we would just as often help our patients get dental work done, land a lease on an apartment, or practice for a job interview. We worked with a women's safe house because once I had seen the wounds of a battered female patient, the thought of sending her back for more of the same made me sick to my stomach. It was, of course, the same sickening feeling that hit me when I realized heroin-addicted patients died because some politicians would not allow provision of methadone treatment, for ideological or populist reasons.

Yet this gut-wrenching feeling is only a starting point for dealing with the difficult issues of addiction. From the beginning it has been clear to me that we also need to work hard on gaining a scientific understanding of this condition. Clearly a better mechanistic understanding of addiction can be expected to offer increasingly effective treatment approaches. But another reason is almost as important. The behaviors of people who compulsively use drugs or alcohol are not only incredibly destructive and self-defeating but also seemingly incomprehensible and scary. Therein lies a big part of the reason the average person so easily distances himself or herself from those with addictive disorders. A better scientific understanding of what makes people become addicted, explained in a way the average person can understand, will help reduce the stigma of addiction. For these reasons, addiction science and addiction medicine offer opportunities to do something that is as practical as it is challenging, important, and gratifying. Yet for all its practicality, the science of addiction is also a window on the fascinating brain functions that make us who we are. This is truly the last frontier of medicine, and a field to consider for every talented medical student, psychologist, or neuroscientist who wants to accomplish something as meaningful as it is interesting.

In this book I will share some of the amazing advances the neuroscience of addiction has made over the years I have been in the field. I will offer a personal take on what addiction is: a malfunction of some of the most fundamental brain circuits that make us tick, and a disease that is not much different from other chronic, relapsing medical conditions. I trust it will be clear what addiction is not: a moral failing, a simple inability to say no, or a condition that can be cured by mystic incantations. As we move between clinical and basic science, it will be clear that there has, finally, been a striking convergence of the two, including an understanding of the major triggers that make people relapse to drug seeking, and the brain mechanisms those triggers engage. We will see that the scientific advances we have already achieved are able to improve, in major ways, the lives of people with addiction, and that they hold out considerable hope for further progress.

It will also be clear, however, that there is a major need to bring together the emerging science of addiction and the world of treatment. I will describe how people with addictive disorders continue to be offered, with great certitude and frequently at great cost, "treatments" that are unsubstantiated by data or already known to be without beneficial effects. Meanwhile, advances that may be modest but have solid scientific support are arrogantly rejected by treatment providers in ways that would cause uproar in other areas of medicine.

A striking example that I will discuss is the medication naltrexone, approved by the Food and Drug Administration (FDA) for alcoholism treatment and supported by extensive evidence but provided only to a tiny fraction of patients who would benefit from it. A broadcast of *Larry King Live* from 2007 illustrates the problem that needs fixing. In the broadcast Susan Ford, at the time chair of the Betty Ford Center in Arizona, debated with my then colleague at the National Institute on Alcohol Abuse and Alcoholism (NIAAA), Mark Willenbring. Ignoring Mark's thorough digest of research data, Ford simply dismissed naltrexone and other anticraving medications as something she and her institution just do not "believe in."

In recent years, attitudes at the Betty Ford Center may have come closer in line with the scientific evidence, but similar attitudes continue to prevent patients from access to life-saving, scientifically well-understood and documented treatments such as methadone and buprenorphine maintenance for heroin addiction.

These attitudes are obviously very troubling for a number of reasons. One is that resources for addiction treatment are scarce. That being the case, it is tragic that the majority of resources are largely wasted on interventions that do not improve meaningful clinical outcomes.

The reasons are not only ideological, but also financial. It is trivial to mention that a criminal hunger for profit fuels the supply of illicit drugs that kill people, and that tremendous efforts are devoted to a "war on drugs" that is aimed at reducing the supply of these drugs to the market. But alcohol is in the aggregate a much greater cause of death and disability than cocaine, heroin, and cannabis are together. Because alcohol is a legal substance, little attention is paid to the fact that the alcohol beverage industry works as hard to maximize profit at the expense of public health as any street-corner drug dealer. For instance, it consistently opposes efforts that have been proven effective at limiting harm from alcohol, such as higher taxes, a monopoly on sales, and limited store hours. Instead the industry favors measures such as education directed at schools and college students—things that may look good but are known to be ineffective.[2]

But the industries that provide people with addictive substances are only one part of the financial ecosystem of addiction. People who develop alcohol and drug problems frequently are taken advantage of twice—first by those who sell them the drugs, then by others who sell them a "cure." There is a whole addiction treatment industry that generates some $34 billion in annual revenue in the United States alone. Much of this industry preys on people made vulnerable by their addiction by peddling exotic interventions with no scientific basis whatsoever as treatments. Even when more reasonable treatment approaches are offered, they may be extremely costly, while outpatient treatments offered at a fraction of the cost would do just as well.

The time has come to bring together the everyday realities of addictive disorders and the emerging science and available evidence. The science is fascinating; the evidence is modestly encouraging. As important as advancing evidence-based treatments, however, is asking the hard questions about the disconnect between what we know and what we do with and for people with addictive disorders. I hope to have triggered enough curiosity for readers to join me on a journey through patient encounters, neural circuits, and price tags. Let's begin.

2

A GROCERY STORE
THAT CLOSED

FRIDAY NIGHT TO Saturday was the most unattractive tour of duty in the psychiatric emergency room of the old mental hospital, keeping doctors and nurses cloistered while everyone else was enjoying weekend pleasures. Weekday shifts did not mess up weekends, so they were more desirable. From noon Saturday through the rest of the weekend, comp time was offered at twice the hours worked, so it quickly accumulated and offset some of the pain of missing out on weekend fun. But the Friday night tours really had no redeeming features. So it should come as no surprise that, being the youngest doctor on staff, I found myself assigned to quite a few of them.

It was one of those Friday nights. The night shift had just taken charge of the small psychiatric emergency room. They were a hardened crew, used to managing not only the patients, who could range from psychotic and violent to depressed and suicidal, but also the young physicians. The shift manager, a nurse in her late fifties with highlighted hair and a generous frame, was an imposing figure to doctors, nursing assistants, and patients alike. She could appear less than caring. "Hi Sven, is it you again?" she might say. "How about you and I chat about those people talking in your head? You know, if we talk for a while, I'm sure you will not need to come in tonight again." But in fact she was not callous at all. She just knew that the patient with chronic schizophrenia would not get better by coming into the psychiatric emergency room, and that this patient's distress could just as well be alleviated by someone listening for a while and then being firm and directive. Over the phone line she could masterfully pick out the patients who really needed to see us because their demons threatened to scare them off the edge of the cliff or for some other reason. "You're in that much pain, huh? You know, sometimes life really is so painful it is amazing people can carry on. But you need to hold on. I promise, it will get better. I know it's hard for you to believe right now, but take my word for it, I've seen this so many times before. It does get better eventually, you hear me? How about I just send out a car so you can come in and talk to our doctor? I have a really good one tonight. Then maybe you can stay with us and try to get your meds adjusted." To this day I am humbled by how experienced nurses like her, with a phone line and a chart as their only source of information, were able to make these difficult calls. When I was much further along in my career, I decided I would give it a try myself, just for the experience. I ended up telling almost every patient who called to come in, flooding the emergency room beyond workable.

The shift manager treated us young doctors much the same way she treated the patients. "Sign here" was her most common comment to us, often without us ever having a chance to talk to the patient or even think about the order we were being asked to sign. Only when I had won her confidence did she start to tell me, one quiet night, about the crazy, inconsistent, or outright dangerous things she had seen done by physicians who were passing through her post on a rotation and could not wait to move on. She spoke passionately about how she viewed herself as an advocate for the patients, with an obligation to protect them from the whims of doctors who, most of the time, were en route to a career somewhere else.

That particular Friday night we received a desperate call from Eric's wife. He was drinking again. Now, a common theme throughout this book is that relapse does not have to be a disaster. As I will discuss, it is an expected element of any chronic disorder such as addiction, much the way it is with hypertension, asthma, or diabetes. It should be approached with calmness, optimism, and a belief that something can be learned from each episode, helping the patient to better manage future challenges. But some cases are different, and I had an unpleasant feeling that Eric's relapse was one of those. He was obese at a level that by itself put him at high risk for major medical complications, and he had an insulin-dependent diabetes that got more out of control with every new episode of drinking. After seeing many patients with catastrophic outcomes, I have learned that my gut feeling is worth paying attention to.

I had seen Eric a couple of times before. This was prior to the era of the modern alcoholism medications. For whatever it was worth, we had suggested that he take Antabuse, but we could not convince him that it would be helpful. At least I had managed to get him seen for a series of sessions by our wonderful social worker. Despite a rheumatoid arthritis that had turned her own hands into painfully twisted stumps—or maybe because of it—she was better than any of us at conveying hope and coaching change. Yet for all her charisma, talk therapy had not done much good in Eric's case, just as it didn't in too many others.

Because of his medical condition, I had a last resort that over several months had kept Eric out of trouble. In those days there was a law on the books that allowed involuntary admission for a patient who, because of ongoing drug or alcohol use, risked severe medical complications or death. Most physicians, I quickly learned, looked the other way rather than invoking that paragraph. They would perhaps consider it if they were dealing with a drug perceived as being really dangerous, such as heroin, abundant in our region. Alcohol problems, however, tended to be the subject of indifference at best.

But I was young and idealistic. After his latest admission, I had told Eric that if he continued to drink despite his diabetes, I would have to write the court papers that would have him locked up to save him from himself. His wife had accompanied him to that visit, and her relief was palpable. Finally someone was going to help. Eric had already told me I was one difficult guy, but he somehow still liked me. He knew I was serious, and he could not afford to be locked up to be dried out. He had a grocery store to run. I wrote a referral to a local clinic for regular checkups, made an agreement that his wife would contact me if it looked like he might be about to fall off the wagon, and parted ways with the couple. I did not hear from them for quite some time and came away with the impression that if I cared, and managed to stand firm, it was perhaps not so hard to do some good. So it was only appropriate that I was working the night, months later, when Eric's wife called. She was crying but was able to convey the seriousness of the situation. Eric was drinking again and had stopped taking his insulin or, worse still, was taking it in a random manner. He had passed out a couple of times already, and it was difficult to know if it was because of low blood sugar, intoxication, or both. He took the phone when I asked to speak to him. Even though I could hear how slurred his speech was, he insisted that he was not drinking.

I asked him to get into a taxi and come in so that we could admit him, detox him, and try to get things on track again. He refused. I said we could send a taxi for him. No luck. After all, there was no need: he was not drinking. Finally I told Eric I would ask the police to bring him in for involuntary admission, said good-bye, and went on to fill out the paperwork.

The scene that followed a few hours later has stuck with me to this very day. The dimly lit corridor of the emergency room. The two police officers. Eric's crying wife. And in the foreground, Eric himself, amazingly enough not at all upset with me. Quite the opposite. He was cheerfully waving to me and saying, "Don't worry, doc. It's all right. I only had a light beer with lunch, that's all." At the same time the nurse, from behind him and over his shoulder, was showing me his breath alcohol level—380 mg/dl, a level close to which a person without profound tolerance is at risk of arrested breathing resulting in death. Eric, meanwhile, managed to walk by his own devices, his large body seemingly only slightly off balance. When the officers left and Eric was being rolled off to the locked intake ward, he kept saying, "It's OK, doc. Just a beer. It's nothing."

Eric was admitted that night and detoxed over the next week, but after that there was little else we could do. The immediate danger that justified the involuntary admission was over. We offered extended residential care, an expensive option we thought in those days was helpful but could choose only in select cases. He was not interested. He went home and died shortly afterward. I cannot remember whether it was a diabetic coma or something else that got him, but I do remember the feeling of being powerless that his wife and I shared after he was gone.

Sometime later, as I was crossing the campus for an all too rare lunch with my father, I looked at the bottom floor of the student apartment building and a sadness came over me. Since my first day of medical school, Eric's grocery store had been a constant—the place students had gone to for milk, cheap noodles, and other essentials. Then there was nothing; groceries would no longer be sold there.

This was one of my early lessons about the destructive force of addiction, the limitlessness of denial, and the insufficiency of the tools medicine had placed at my disposal. Obviously, countless more lessons would follow. Maybe one reason this one stuck with me is that it freed me of some of my innocence and naïveté. But it also captured several elements from which a journey into the landscape of addiction should start, each of which we will revisit in detail along the way: that addiction makes people continue to use a drug even if they know it causes them severe harm and is likely ultimately to cost them their life. That nice people who might be perfectly able to contribute to society still may end up using drugs until they die. That the potential for denial, both from the patient and from everyone else, until it is too late exceeds most people's imagination. That trying to talk the addict out of drug use is challenging at best. And that trying to force the person to quit, even if feasible, is not very helpful other than in the shortest of terms.

The story of my encounter with Eric also says something about a drug that may not receive the attention it merits. When I ask students what addictive drug they consider to be the most damaging, I get different answers. Some say heroin, particularly if they have paid attention to how deadly it can be for the individual overdosing.[1] Others say cocaine, which is widely associated with violent crime, ravaged inner cities, murderous cartels, and the whole war on drugs. Others still say crystal meth, which is more potent than cocaine and so should command considerable respect. Some, not entirely unreasonably, say nicotine, citing data such as those indicating that among people who have tried this drug, the proportion found to be addicted is higher than for any other addictive substance.[2]

Few students say that alcohol is the most damaging drug. Yet data from the World Health Organization show that among addictive drugs, the toll of death and disease caused by alcohol use is surpassed only by that caused by nicotine. And nicotine is a special case because it does not cause much harm itself. After all, we know that a skin patch that delivers nicotine is reasonably safe. It is instead the use of tobacco products that causes nicotine-associated harm. In that respect, alcohol addiction is much more similar to illicit drugs and causes more harm than any of those.

One way of calculating the harm associated with a condition, widely accepted across different areas of medicine, is to sum up the number of *quality-adjusted life years* lost owing to that condition. If life expectancy is seventy years and someone dies at forty, clearly thirty years were lost, adjusted or not. But if someone instead dies at age sixty after having had, on average, a 50 percent disability for twenty years, the loss is twenty quality-adjusted years. By this measure, harm from alcohol use amounts to about 10 percent of total disability-adjusted life years lost in industrialized countries.[3]

It might be argued that the analysis above is insufficient, and I would tend to agree. The measure of disability described is based on the harm caused to the individual using the drug. Clearly, however, addictive drugs also cause extensive harm to others, through crime, accidents, lost productivity, broken families, and other social costs. The former adviser to the British government on matters of addiction, David Nutt of London's Imperial College, concluded that in aggregate, the harm to self and others inflicted by alcohol exceeds that caused by heroin or cocaine.[4] Although by no means undisputed, this analysis captures something important.

Finally, one might argue that the harm measures from these different sources, while telling us something about alcohol, do not necessarily say much about alcohol addiction. After all, alcohol consumption is widespread among people who are not addicted. But while it is indisputable that only a minority of people who consume alcohol are addicted, and that people can be harmed by alcohol without being addicted, it is also a fact that alcohol consumption in the population is markedly skewed: about 10 percent of the population consumes more than half of all alcohol consumed.[5] Thus an overwhelming proportion of alcohol-related disability is due to what I will call alcohol addiction and hereafter equate with "alcoholism." This condition affects more than 10 percent of the population at some point in the United States and other industrialized countries.[6] Alcohol addiction is a prototype for a group of conditions characterized by continued use despite adverse consequences. While there are certainly important differences, the lessons learned about alcoholism are therefore helpful for understanding addiction in general. So before moving on, I will spend some time describing what addiction is and is not, with much of the focus on alcohol addiction.

3

AN ENTITY IN ITS OWN RIGHT

Anyone concerned with treating drinking problems must find that his patients often tell him more than is in the textbooks. Each tells a different story, but there are also repeated patterns. Much of the varied experience that is recounted can be interpreted as the patient's astute observation of the alcohol dependence syndrome—a condition certainly far better described by the average alcoholic than in any book.

—G. EDWARDS AND M. M. GROSS, "ALCOHOL DEPENDENCE" (1976)

D EPENDENCE, ABUSE, substance use disorders, addiction. There are so many terms, used by professionals and laypeople alike, that do not necessarily have a clear meaning. Each attempts to capture substance use that is harmful, but drugs can be harmful in different ways. To build an understanding of the kind of substance use that gives rise to clinical problems, we need to know what we are talking about.

So let's step back a little. A desire to chemically alter brain function and the mind states it produces is probably as old as humankind itself. We know that the ancient Greeks considered the knowledge of how to ferment grape juice into wine to be a gift from the god Bacchus and held annual celebrations to commemorate it. An even more striking example comes from the Russian tundra, where temperatures never rise high enough to allow fermentation of alcoholic beverages. The nomads of these lands devoted precious time and energy to seeking out mushrooms containing substances that, when ingested, produce a state of intoxication dominated by confusion, a dry mouth, and constipation.[1] A feature of this drug is that it is excreted in the urine without being chemically degraded. Because of that, it is said that toward the end of a long winter, a measure of an adult male's urine could be exchanged for a reindeer cow, which must have represented a fortune.

Clearly the amount of effort an individual is willing to expend to obtain a drug tells us something important about its motivational value. We will see that this applies to humans and animals alike, allowing scientists, under controlled conditions in the laboratory, to assess motivation to obtain a drug. I hasten to say that the example of the mushrooms, while colorful, is not the most didactic. The nomads did not have access to other drugs. When alternatives are present, neither people nor animals will in fact work for this particular drug class. That observation, however, may be useful in itself. It tells us that the motivational value of a drug, or, for that matter, of anything, is not absolute or constant. Instead it is determined by many things. Among these, the choices available to the individual at the time are an important environmental variable.[2]

Little has changed in modern times. Mind-altering or "psychotropic" drug effects remain sought after. The means to achieve these effects vary and are in part determined by culture and availability, illustrating another set of important environmental variables. Many efforts to reduce drug use by educating the public are based on the assumption that substance use is a consequence of ignorance. For the most part, that is simply not the case. In modern Western countries, where the public is better educated on the potential consequences of alcohol use than ever in the history of our species, between 50 and 90 percent of the adult population consumes alcohol, and a significant minority develop problems because of their use. In other contemporary societies, various formulations of the hemp species *Cannabis sativa* or *indica*, or the opium poppy, *Papaver somniferum*, remain in widespread use. And nicotine use is on the rise in the third world as people become more affluent and better educated. It seems clear that whatever these drugs do, large numbers of people are willing to take them, even though they know the risks. What accounts for this willingness, of course, are the pharmacological, mind-altering properties of the substances that most people are after.

But here we must pause. Most people enjoy the relaxed social inhibitions that result from having a couple of drinks at a cocktail party. Most people who sample cocaine experience euphoria. Yet most people who try these drugs will not get in trouble because of their substance use. This is a fundamental issue when we try to understand the people who *do* develop problems, get sick, and in many cases die as a consequence of substance use. No matter which drug we look at, only a minority of people using it will develop medical or psychological problems. Meanwhile, a majority will be able to occasionally sample the same drug, or engage in intermittent recreational use over decades, without measurable harm.

Work published by James Anthony, at the time at Johns Hopkins University in Baltimore, uses data from two large epidemiological studies, and provides a perspective on this phenomenon.[3] These studies examined large numbers of people from the general population and focused on those who had ever used potentially addictive substances or who were still active users, respectively. Anthony and his colleagues applied standard clinical diagnostic criteria to determine the fraction of those people who would qualify for a diagnosis of "dependence," the official diagnostic category (defined later in this chapter). Among active users, the numbers ranged between 8 and 18 percent. The exception was nicotine, for which 34 percent of active users qualified for a diagnosis of dependence. As mentioned in the previous chapter, this does not necessarily imply the counterintuitive conclusion that is sometimes drawn from these data—that nicotine is more addictive than all other drugs. The barriers to obtaining and using cocaine are clearly much higher than those to obtaining nicotine. The important message here is that even among active users of the most addictive drugs, such as cocaine or heroin, only a minority develop a particularly destructive relationship with the drug. And in most cases, those who do develop this relationship take a long time—years or decades—to do so.

These observations in turn raise an important and much debated question. Is there really any important difference between people who develop a destructive relationship with a drug and those who do not? Is there, as some would have it, a line, however bright, the crossing of which signifies an important transition and justifies distinguishing those who have crossed it from those who have not? Or is all substance use in principle equal, and harmful in varying degrees that depend only on the amounts used and the social, economic, or medical circumstances of the individual?

The medical profession comes down firmly on one side of this fundamental question. Someone is either healthy or ill, and in the latter case there had better be a diagnostic label for the disease or the doctor may not get reimbursed for its treatment. Indeed, the World Health Organization (WHO), in the tenth revision of its *International Classification of Diseases and Health Problems* (ICD-10) from 1992,[4] defines a "substance dependence syndrome"[5] that is similar to that described in the classic paper by Edwards and Gross quoted at the outset of this chapter. This syndrome is described as a cluster of physiological, behavioral, and cognitive phenomena in which the use of a substance or a class of substances takes on a much higher priority for an individual than other behaviors that once had greater value. A central characteristic of the dependence syndrome is said to be a strong, often overpowering desire to obtain and use the psychoactive drug, which for the rest of this book I will refer to as "craving." Dependence, as defined by the WHO, refers to both psychological and physical phenomena. The criteria refer to "psychological dependence" as the experience of impaired control over drinking or drug use. "Physiological" or simply "physical" dependence is used to denote tolerance and withdrawal symptoms.[6]

Well, the doctor is always right, so what else is there to say? Quite a bit, of course, as anyone familiar with the history and the controversies of this field over the years well knows. For starters, the medical profession cannot have the final say on this subject. Although doctors devote more time than they may realize to treating medical consequences of drug and alcohol use, they are not a major presence in treating whatever it is that makes people engage in this use in the first place. For better and worse, psychologists, counselors, and mutual-help groups play a much greater role than doctors in treating people with substance use problems. Increased involvement of the medical profession is certainly needed, in particular as medications become an increasingly important component of an effective treatment package. But there will always be a major need for the contributions from other professions, and all of us will always need to establish an alliance and a dialogue with the patients themselves. So leaving scientific and philosophical issues aside, we have an important need for a common language, simply from the standpoint of clinical practicality. In seeking this common language, it is necessary to understand that for many sociologists and psychologists, a categorical view such as that espoused by the medical profession is quite foreign and problematic. A philosophical discussion of this fundamental yet controversial issue can quickly become involved, and both sides have valid arguments. In the end, my view is that whether there is a difference between people who develop a destructive relationship with a drug and those who do not needs to be determined by clinical utility. If there are certain characteristics that tend to occur together in people with particular treatment needs, or in whom similar mechanisms are at play that could be targeted by current or future treatments, then it is practical to have a specifically labeled category (or group of categories) for those people.

The fundamental question we are dealing with here breaks down into at least three parts. First, are there systematic and meaningful differences between people with a "dependence syndrome" or some similarly labeled condition and those without it? Second, what is the most appropriate label for such a condition or group of conditions, should we decide that they make up a meaningful category? Third, should the categories we ultimately define be viewed as medical conditions or, for short, "diseases"?

With a number of important caveats, the answer to the first question is most likely "yes." There are indeed a number of common features, recognized by patients, family members, and clinicians alike, that are shared by large numbers of people who are harmed by their alcohol or drug use. With the help of the WHO, I have already started outlining those features above. Are they useful to delineate a clinically relevant group among all the individuals that ever use a substance? Perhaps somewhat surprisingly, basic science has recently started to shed some interesting light on this question.

Almost all drugs that are abused by humans are also self-administered by experimental animals.[7] The classical model involves placing a rat or mouse in a box with levers that can be pressed or buttons that can be poked using the nose. When the animal presses a lever or pokes a button, a pump is started and delivers a dose of a drug as a reward—through an intravenous catheter in the case of cocaine or heroin, or into a little cup in the case of alcohol. Animals readily lever press or nose poke for drugs such as cocaine, heroin, or alcohol, so these drugs can be called rewarding. Or at least, as a stricter experimental psychologist would probably prefer, they are reinforcing, meaning that the behavior that led their delivery becomes more frequent than in the absence of the outcome.

But here is a challenge. Almost all rats or mice will readily and within days self-administer heroin or cocaine. Alcohol takes a bit longer, in part because animals initially dislike its taste, and also because it takes longer for the brain effects caused by alcohol to be experienced, making it harder for the animal to learn that they are a consequence of its behavior. Nevertheless, within a few weeks, most rats and mice will self-administer alcohol as well.

Self-administration, studied in this way, has become the standard model by which scientists study brain mechanisms through which abused drugs work and test medications that might be helpful in treating their use. But doesn't that seem odd? I just went over human research indicating that, by clinical diagnostic criteria, only a minority of active users of any substance will develop substance dependence, and that this takes them many years, sometimes decades. Are the diagnostic criteria arbitrary after all?

Probably not. A few years back, two different laboratories, one in France and one in the United Kingdom, evaluated some of the core features defined by the established clinical diagnostic criteria for drug dependence in animal experiments that used the self-administration model in a particularly clever way.[8] In one of these studies, which took note of the fact that clinical dependence takes time to develop, rats were first allowed to self-administer cocaine for an unusually long period of time. A month of forced abstinence followed the self-administration phase. Finally, after the forced abstinence, the animals were tested for relapse to drug seeking, using a model I will describe in more detail in a coming chapter. Although all the animals had been given the same access to cocaine during the self-administration phase, about one in five showed an interesting constellation of features. While still in the self-administration phase, they had been particularly persistent in their drug seeking, nose poking even during breaks in the sessions, when the drug was not available. It was as if they could not stop themselves. They had also continued their drug taking even when this led to adverse consequences, in this case a mild electric shock that made other animals stop their self-administration. Finally, they had exhibited the highest motivation to obtain the drug, measured as the maximal number of nose pokes they were willing to make to obtain a dose of cocaine. The animals showing these three characteristics were also those that were particularly prone to relapse after the month of abstinence. With about one in five rats showing this special pattern of drug use, the fraction was clearly similar to that seen in human epidemiological studies. This pattern of drug use could be called compulsive because the animals no longer seemed able to flexibly change their behavior the way their fellow subjects were.

If compulsive drug use, as characterized by these features, is a hallmark of clinically important substance use syndromes, then it would seem clear that these syndromes are primarily conditions of malfunctioning motivational machinery and control of behavior, reflecting processes in the brain, even though what brings the patient to the doctor may be a cirrhotic liver or some other damaged organ.[9] In fact, the most striking observation from many years of working with people who seek treatment for alcohol or drug problems is that their motivational machinery somehow seems broken. The job of this sophisticated brain circuitry is to guide behavior, so that a person can be reasonably successful in the pursuit of his or her goals and, if one believes in such a thing, of happiness.[10] As we know from our own lives, this machinery is by no means perfect. But it generally does not make simple, disastrous blunders when better choices are readily and immediately available. Yet that is what happens over and over again for people like Eric in the previous chapter. Contrary to widespread public belief, this is not because of any moral flaw in these people or a lack of understanding on their part. When asked, no patient I ever met really valued getting drunk over having a job or a home. Yet they would easily and repeatedly lose both these things and then some for an opportunity to get drunk or high. Likewise, unless severely depressed,[11] patients don't want to die when a decent life is an option. Yet like Eric, many patients continue to engage in substance use despite knowing full well that deteriorating health and ultimately death are likely to result.

Although this inability to steer behavior toward desired goals is at the core of compulsive substance use, that process plays out over years, and assessing it can easily become rather subjective in the individual case. The clinician needs to know whether compulsive drug use is manifested by some simpler features that can be observed here and now, and be less subject to debate. The patients who over the years engage in substance use that takes them far away from their goals do seem to share a number of simpler, clinically meaningful features that pass the utility test. None of these features on its own is necessary or sufficient to identify people with compulsive drug use, but when enough features are present, we can be fairly certain.

One characteristic is simply that alcohol or drug use escalates over time, a feature that has been replicated in experimental animals.[12] As escalation occurs, it takes more and more drug to get the same buzz but also to become impaired—the classic signs of developing tolerance. Patients notice that when they stop, they become anxious, shaky, or miserable in other ways—withdrawal syndromes that are in part different for each drug but tend to be a mirror image of the acute drug effects. Patients attempt to limit the quantities of drug that are used but repeatedly find that, to no one's surprise except their own, instead of having just one glass of wine with dinner they end up consuming every bottle available, falling asleep on the floor, and throwing up on the carpet. To control intake better, they impose periods of abstinence, often in the hope that they will be able to resume controlled alcohol or drug use after having stayed sober or drug free long enough. But they can't. The next attempt to engage in social, controlled use that the rest of us can easily manage ends with the same rapid escalation of intake and consumption of much more than was intended. These are all objective, observable facts. The last characteristic may be more open to debate because it relies on subjective reports from patients. But after seeing heroin addicts who stayed clean for years become distressed and sweat profusely at the sight of needles and syringes, I have become convinced that craving—the persistent and overpowering desire to resume drug use even after prolonged abstinence—is as real as any of the other features and is what drives continued substance use despite adverse consequences.

Right here is the core of most attempts to capture a clinical syndrome that denotes an important relationship between a drug and the individual using it. In various constellations, this syndrome is what the WHO and the American Psychiatric Association have attempted to define in their diagnostic catalogs under labels such as "substance dependence" or "substance use disorder." Whatever the name and the exact diagnostic criteria, what we are trying to capture is a condition associated with extensive medical, psychological, and social consequences. As I write these words, I catch myself because I am reminded that I have somehow lost my way—what I just wrote is hiding the fact that we are dealing with a set of conditions that make people sick, make them desperately sad and anxious, can even kill them, disrupt their families, harm their children physically and emotionally, and cause losses to productivity in the trillions—not to mention all the losses due to drug-related crimes. So yes, there is a category worth distinguishing and having a label for. But before moving on to the issue whether dependence, substance use disorder, or something else is the best label for this important category, we need to branch out and deal with two other categories that are frequently discussed.

First, many people indiscriminately refer to the use of illicit drugs or the problematic use of alcohol as "abuse." In a seemingly more precise definition, this label has also been used as a clinical diagnosis. The idea is that if someone did not qualify for a diagnosis of dependence but still used alcohol or drugs to the point of failing to fulfill obligations in the workplace or in family life, or if one got in trouble through fights or risky behaviors under the influence of a substance, one had a condition that could be called abuse.

Extensive research has shown that this label is essentially meaningless. People with this type of substance-related problem can be found anywhere along the spectrum of substance use severity. Some have what we have so far referred to as dependence. Others have nothing of the kind but may, for instance, live in environments where norm breaking, fights, or other dangerous behaviors are not contained by stable social structures. Most people receive a "diagnosis" of abuse because of a single behavior, such as being caught driving while intoxicated. Unless this is associated with compulsive substance use, I don't think it is a medical diagnosis. Yes, it is dangerous, irresponsible behavior, but as a physician I do not have any more tools to help out with it than any other sensible adult does. Abuse is simply not a clinically meaningful concept. Large epidemiological studies, such as the National Epidemiological Survey on Alcohol and Related Conditions (NESARC) sponsored by the NIAAA, strongly support this conclusion. As a consequence, the latest edition of the diagnostic manual from the American Psychiatric Association has eliminated abuse as a diagnosis.

Second, it should be obvious that neither substance dependence nor abuse criteria capture everyone who is harmed by their alcohol or drug use. This is particularly important to consider for alcohol because it is so widely used, and because it is such a nasty, unusually toxic drug. It is, for instance, possible for someone who is still in control of their alcohol consumption to develop severe medical problems from alcohol. If a patient has a certain genetic predisposition and has not been told that consuming half a bottle of wine daily with dinner is a major factor behind his hypertension, he could easily end up receiving antihypertensive treatment for decades, until he ultimately develops congestive heart failure, yet never be the wiser. So it is important to recognize and identify a category that we may call hazardous alcohol use, which does not necessarily imply compulsivity. This concept is tremendously helpful in reducing medical problems caused by alcohol use in the general population. We will revisit it when discussing behavioral treatments. For now, let me just mention that if a good family physician assessed our patient's alcohol consumption and told him about the connection, the patient would in most cases be able to change his behavior, with dramatic improvements in health outcomes as a result.[13] After all, as I said, we are in pursuit of happiness. There is very little happiness to be found in daily intake of a beta blocker, or becoming unable to climb a flight of stairs. Yes, old habits die hard. Yes, it is a struggle. But ultimately, unless they have developed compulsive drug use, most people are able to change their behavior to achieve their goals. This is fundamentally different from Eric and his fellow patients.

This brings us back to compulsive use, and the special relationship between the person and the drug we have so far delineated as substance dependence syndrome. By now I hope to have made a convincing argument that it is, after all, justified to reserve a category for people with compulsive use—Eric's kind of relationship with a substance. There are nevertheless some important caveats to consider.

First, if such a category should be delineated, it should be done knowing that we have only imperfect tools to do so. There is no blood test, brain scan, or other objective measure. The diagnostic criteria are all reasonable and reflect a great deal of clinical wisdom. But we have some ways to go. When scientists ask questions of the general population, they find that about 12 percent of Americans qualify for ever having had a diagnosis of alcohol dependence, and about 4 percent receive this diagnosis at the time of being assessed. The numbers are typically twice as high for men as for women. Adding people with dependence on other drugs does not greatly increase the 4 percent number, indicating both that vastly more people have alcohol problems than drug problems and that drug problems frequently occur in people who also have alcohol problems.[14]

Wait a moment. Yes, drug and alcohol problems are terribly common, but are they really this common—one in twenty-five adults with a serious substance use diagnosis at any given time? I'm not so sure. The fact is that a majority of these people never seek or receive any treatment. In many cases that is clearly because access to treatment and insurance coverage are sorely lacking. But it is equally clear that in many other cases, these are people who continue to live their lives without negative medical or social consequences. That makes one wonder just how good a job our diagnostic criteria do at capturing what we are after. It turns out that it's probably not so good if applied outside of a clinical setting. When people in the general population received a diagnosis of ever having had alcohol dependence and then were reinterviewed five years later, two-thirds of the women and one-third of the men no longer received the same diagnosis.[15] Remember, this was about *ever* having had alcohol dependence. So unless a fairy had allowed these people to relive their lives and change already lived history, the real number of people with a diagnosis simply could not have decreased.

The situation becomes very different, however, if we add one more requirement. Among people who in the first round had received a diagnosis *and* sought treatment, almost all, or nine out of ten, still qualified for the diagnosis five years later. Clearly, as indicated by Edwards and Gross in the quote that opened this chapter, the patients know something about their alcoholism that the textbooks do not know. They tell us about it when they seek treatment. Accordingly, other studies indicate that treatment-seeking alcoholics and those who qualify for the same diagnosis but never seek treatment largely come from two different populations. To emphasize that distinction, I frequently refer to "clinical alcoholism" when discussing the former group.

Second, a single category may seem justified by common clinical features, but as we will find in the coming chapters, that is in part something we could call the clinician's fallacy. Clinical alcoholism and corresponding conditions related to the use of other drugs are what I call end-stage diseases. To explain this concept I could use as an example the diagnosis of kidney failure, with which most people are familiar. Although this diagnosis sounds precise enough, the people who receive it in fact represent the final stage in one of many different processes, with diabetes and hypertension being the most common. Similarly, there are many different trajectories through which a patient can arrive at a diagnosis of alcohol dependence. While these patients may share clinically important features here and now, it is likely that the underlying biology is very different. In one case, for instance, someone rapidly arrived at his diagnosis because of gene variants that made him tolerate large amounts of alcohol without becoming impaired, perhaps also associated with impulsive behavior and getting a strong kick out of alcohol intake. In another case, alcohol dependence evolved over the course of decades as a result of gradually increasing alcohol consumption, with reduction of social anxiety as the main motivational driver. If, as is likely, the underlying biology is different in these cases, then maybe the response to treatments will be as well. So while, for lack of better alternatives, we may settle for a single diagnosis for these patients for now, we should constantly be on the lookout to pick apart or deconstruct this category into biologically more meaningful subgroups. More about that later.

Having come this far, we are ready to ask, at last, what might be the most appropriate name for the category, or group of categories, I have so far delineated. I have already given away the name that for decades was the official one, "dependence," used by Edwards and Gross above. I love that classic paper, and its message that patients with alcohol problems know something important about their condition that we may not be able to find in a textbook. But the choice of the word "dependence" is terrible. Outside a limited circle of scientists and specialized clinicians, dependence is typically interpreted as physical dependence, characterized by tolerance and withdrawal. As a result, laypeople and professionals alike continue to view these two phenomena as integral to clinically significant substance use disorders. And yet we know now that compulsive drug use reflects pathology of motivational brain circuitry, not the shakes of coming off alcohol. Dependence, in the physiological sense most commonly given to it, is neither necessary nor sufficient as an ingredient in a substance use disorder.

The failure to make that distinction for decades has been doubly problematic. Here are illustrations of the two sides of that coin: On one hand, Δ^9-THC, the active ingredient of marijuana, is eliminated by the body so slowly that it essentially provides a built-in taper, masking the expression of withdrawal and frequently leading people to believe that cannabinoids are somehow less addictive[16] than other classes of drugs. On the other hand, even though the vast majority of benzodiazepine-treated patients do not develop addiction, their predictable needs for dose increases over the long term, and the emergence of accentuated symptoms on discontinuation has given rise to an entire cottage industry of "taper treatments." Based on this misconception, patients with debilitating anxiety disorders frequently have their successful treatments discontinued to address their presumed benzodiazepine dependence. Worse still, the mixup has allowed ideologues generally opposed to antidepressant treatments to claim that these are addictive, too, because—similar to antihypertensive drugs—there is a discontinuation syndrome.

Addressing this confusion is long overdue. It is effectively done using the term "addiction," which focuses on the core motivational problems that lead to compulsive substance use that continues despite adverse consequences. This issue remains contentious, with one argument being that the term carries a stigma. The latest edition of the diagnostic manual published by the

American Psychiatric Association tries to square this circle by calling the chapter in which these conditions are described "Substance Use and Addictive Disorders" but avoiding the addiction label in the specific, individual diagnostic names. Instead there is for each drug a single category, such as "alcohol use disorder," of varying severity. I have great sympathy for the concerns about stigma. But a better way of addressing that issue is working against stigma through improved scientific understanding, improved treatments, and education of the public and policy makers. In the absence of that, inventing new names for the same thing may not solve anything. Before we know it, the new name will be equally stigmatizing.

So addiction it is. But is addiction a disease?

4

A CHRONIC,
RELAPSING DISORDER

IT WAS 1997. I had just been appointed director of a large, newly created addiction medicine service in the Swedish capital city of Stockholm. We had a staff of about four hundred, close to a hundred inpatient beds, an emergency room of our own in the city center, and clinics scattered across several locations in the most drug-infested part of the region. There was just one problem. Although we were affiliated with the famous Karolinska Institute, we had no idea what we were doing.

The patients were mostly poor, severely addicted, and socially marginalized people. Many were homeless or, as I would soon learn, in various stages of a homelessness progression that is not as clear as people with real homes tend to think. Sometimes patients would show up in our emergency room with severe withdrawal, delirium tremens, seizures, or overdoses. On other occasions it would be malnutrition, dehydration, or a kind of general medical derangement that is hard to pin down to a specific diagnostic code yet is probably a more important clinical finding than many well-defined conditions. And then there was the steady stream of people who spoke of being depressed and said they contemplated suicide. Sometimes, it was clear, they faked it to gain admission, when the night got too cold and the shelters were full. Could we really blame them? On other occasions they truly meant it right there and then but were fine after a night in a bed, a meal, and some talking. But I also knew that these were patients whose rates of completed suicide were about five times higher than those of the general population.

Events had thrown me into the job far too young and utterly unprepared. I had arrived at the Karolinska only two years earlier, fresh out of my psychiatry residency. Psychiatry and addiction had always fascinated me, but my research training was in basic neuropharmacology, in which I had obtained a doctorate and then spent two crazy, wonderful years as a postdoctoral fellow with George Koob at the Scripps Research Institute in La Jolla, California. When I was recruited to the Karolinska, it was to continue my basic science work while slowly building a small clinical research unit. I expected to be learning on the job and initially felt insecure and intimidated. A year into it, my anxieties had begun to ease. Having originally trained in a charming, medieval university town with a population of about 100,000 and little if any serious crime, I had been concerned that my clinical training might leave me unprepared to deal with the severe drug, alcohol, and crime problems of the big city. But the patients I had been seeing had been reasonably socially stable, with medical problems that for the most part seemed manageable. I had been able to start building the research program just like I had planned, train staff, obtain research grants, teach, and settle into a comfortable existence in academic medicine.

And then the hospital system decided to reshuffle everything. Several services were put together into fewer, larger departments in a way that seemed to serve only two purposes: to disguise large cutbacks in services for an already underserved patient category, and to give some bureaucrats power. I tried to work within the system, even as my best nurses one after another abandoned ship, but in the end I found that I couldn't. I recall sitting in my office late one afternoon, after the last patient appointment, leafing through a medical journal and seeing an ad for a director's job on the other side of town. I remember leaving it there, with the page open, for several days before the next peak of frustration prompted me to write the application letter, mostly as a way to release the frustration. George Koob, who not only had remained a great mentor but also become a good friend, came by for a talk at the Karolinska just as I was thinking whether I should accept the job offer; he told me, in his characteristically blunt way,

"Markus, there is one biologically undeniable truth. It is always better to be in control than not."

So I held on to the best thing the old hospital had offered, which was a beautiful, warmhearted nurse who was soon to become my wife, left everything else, and took the job—only to discover that rather than being in control, I was confronted with an entirely new and previously unimaginable level of feeling powerless. Yes, I could make many more decisions about what treatments to provide and how. But what were the right decisions to make? I was completely, utterly out of my depth.

The fundamental problem was this: We could—and did—debate which patients should be admitted, or how long a detox should be. We could argue over whether detox medications should be used,[1] and if so, which ones, at what doses, and for how long. After that, we could do all in our power to engage social workers and get them to help with discharge planning and organizing funding for treatment at a residential facility for twenty-eight days or maybe longer. This last step was viewed as the ultimate success, harder and harder to achieve as public finances worsened. But it took just a small step back from the day-to-day management, and a look with a slightly dispassionate eye, to see that the hard work of our staff made little significant dent in the disease process of addiction, which meanwhile was killing our patients. This is not to negate the value of a bed and a meal for a homeless, hungry addict. It is not to understate the power of a kind word or someone being ready to listen and take a person's anguish seriously, even when it is expressed in the middle of the night, through intoxication, and by someone who does not necessarily smell nice. But as a physician, I wanted to make a difference. To take the Hippocratic oath in reverse, I wanted to comfort always, treat often, and preferably also cure sometimes.

It was clear to me that at best we were providing comfort. And I saw that even that was frequently challenging for our staff. Every relapse was taken as a sign either that the patient was not motivated or that we were powerless to change the course of addiction. Over the years, as they saw little of their efforts pay off, some treatment providers quit for less frustrating jobs, while others became hardened, jaded, and seemingly uncaring. We clearly had to change our ways or would continue to burn through our most valuable asset: our staff's compassion and desire to help.

I realized that I was immersed in something quite different from other areas of medicine I had experience with, such as my second love, endocrinology. Evidence-based medicine had by then transformed clinical practice almost everywhere. The latest advances might not be implemented as fast as they should be anywhere, but a young physician could for the most part assume that clinical practice was based on data from controlled studies that showed measurable benefits for patients from specific clinical interventions. Here, I realized, it was quite possible that we were using considerable resources without helping patients with outcomes that mattered. The bitter divisions between different schools of thought alone were enough to show that we couldn't all be practicing based on available evidence. And there was a clear possibility that some of our ways made things worse, not better.

In what little time there was between managing staff, budgets, and patients, haggling with politicians over funding, and trying to be a good enough father for our first child, I read as much as I could. Throughout my career one simple principle has helped me more than anything else, both as a scientist and as a physician: if you don't know what you are doing, quickly find someone who does, and emulate their approach. Every science class should start with a reading of a single sentence by Sir Isaac Newton: "If I saw further than other men, it was because I stood on the shoulders of giants." Clinical medicine is not much different.

I still didn't know exactly what I was doing, but after a while a couple of things seemed clear. Reading the literature was one thing, but we could not just read our way to improving our methods. That would have required me, or someone like me, to integrate the published scientific reports and tell our staff what changes in practice the weight of the evidence implied. Even if I had felt capable of doing that, which I did not, this approach was not likely to get staff onboard, enthusiastic, and past their ideologically driven convictions. To them it would just be another voice articulating a belief, among other voices competing for their attention. But perhaps we could get people out of their entrenched positions if we could do the journey together, in a literal sense. Perhaps we could go on an expedition to a place where clinical needs guided the science, where the science guided the way clinical work was done, and where we might be able to absorb a culture as much as specific knowledge.

The list of places we were able to identify seemed surprisingly short, although at the time I assumed that was because I just did not know the field well enough. I wrote two people I had never met but whose names often appeared on research papers that were as interesting and scientifically stringent as they were relevant for clinical issues of addiction medicine: Charles P. O'Brien and Tom McLellan at the University of Pennsylvania Treatment Research Center in Philadelphia. To my amazement, Chuck, as I soon learned he was called by the entire field, quickly answered, welcomed us, and had someone put together a program for us. It was unheard of to take a whole group of nurse managers on a trip abroad and pay for it out of hospital funds. But I asked that someone show me what regulations we would be breaking, and no one could come up with any. I guess this was one of those situations where being in control indeed was better than not. In Philadelphia we stayed at the cheapest possible hotel on Chestnut Street, the elevator only worked intermittently, and even some of the more hardnosed nurses turned pale when shots were heard in the neighborhood one night.

But it was all worth it: we were in for a treat. To hear Chuck tell the story of how his team discovered naltrexone, the first modern alcoholism medication, was enough to make the visit worthwhile, and I will revisit that story in some detail later. But it was Tom McLellan, in cowboy boots, getting up on the table and explaining the concept of addiction as a chronic, relapsing disease that probably made the greatest impression on our nursing staff.

> So you have a patient with hypertension. You give him a beta blocker, and his blood pressure comes down. Everyone says, "Look, treatment works!" Then for some reason the patient decides to stop the medication. Within weeks, blood pressure is out of control again. Everybody says, "Didn't we tell you—this treatment definitely works, and the patient really needs it!" Now, instead, you have a patient with alcohol addiction. The patient goes into treatment, stops drinking, and improves in every aspect of his life.

Then treatment is discontinued. After a while the patient starts using alcohol again, and things fall apart. At which time family members, the patient's employer and friends all say, "Didn't we know it. Alcoholics really are hopeless. And treatment is a waste of money. People just relapse." Doesn't this all strike you as a bit odd?

The message was one to which we had not previously given much thought. Addiction is inherently a chronic, relapsing disease, not much different from diseases we already have successful management models for, such as hypertension, diabetes, or asthma. Similar to those diseases, the risk for developing addiction has a strong genetic component. Likewise, the development and course of addiction are determined by an intricate interplay among genetic risk factors, environmental influences, and behavioral choices. Addiction cannot currently be cured but can be managed with a degree of success that is sufficient to allow patients to live a good life. If not managed, on the other hand, it disables, kills, and leads to costs and suffering that are hard to fathom. In none of these aspects does addiction differ from other common, complex illnesses of a chronic relapsing nature. Yet for these conditions, long-term disease management that combines pharmacological and behavioral approaches is an undisputed norm, and success is hardly assessed by the number of people completely cured of their ailment. At the same time, we continue to debate whether addiction really is a medical condition, focus on short-term fixes such as detoxification or twenty-eight-day residential programs, see anything other than complete abstinence as a failure, and frequently view the harm caused by addiction as self-inflicted.

A couple of years after our visit to Philadelphia, in 2000, Tom McLellan, Chuck O'Brien, and several other leaders in the field of addiction research forcefully laid out this tragic paradox in a paper in a top medical journal.[2] They started by noting that the effects of addiction[3] on society have helped shape a widely held view that addiction is primarily a social problem, not a health problem. They then examined evidence that addiction is in fact indistinguishable from chronic medical illnesses. They reviewed the scientific literature and compared the role of genetic and environmental factors, disease mechanisms, and treatment outcomes such as adherence to treatment and relapse between addiction, on one hand, and type 2 diabetes mellitus, hypertension, and asthma, on the other. They found that genetic risk factors, personal choice, and environmental factors are comparably involved in the etiology and course of all these disorders. Furthermore, just like consumption of an unhealthful diet produces lasting cardiovascular changes in diabetes, heavy alcohol or drug use produces significant and lasting changes in brain chemistry and function. Despite widespread perceptions to the contrary, effective medications are available for treating several addictions, such as those for nicotine, alcohol, or opiates. Medication adherence and relapse rates are very similar in addictive disorders and the other illnesses with which the comparison was made.

A fundamental problem, the authors concluded, is that addiction generally has largely been treated as if it were an acute illness. Their review instead showed that, similar to the other chronic relapsing illnesses, longterm care strategies of medication management and continued monitoring are the ones that produce lasting benefits. Because of this, addiction should be insured, treated, and evaluated like any other chronic illness. This, they stated, stands in stark contrast with the public view that drug dependence is primarily a social problem that requires interdiction and law enforcement, rather than being a health problem that requires prevention and treatment, a view that many physicians apparently share. Most physicians still fail even to screen for alcohol or drug use during routine examinations, viewing such screening efforts as a waste of time. A survey of general practice physicians and nurses indicated that most believed no available medical or health care interventions would be appropriate or effective in treating addiction.

McClellan and his coauthors noted that 40 to 60 percent of patients treated for alcohol or other drug addiction indeed return to active substance use within a year following treatment discharge. They outlined two distinct possibilities to account for this fact, with different implications. On one hand, it is possible that these disappointing results indeed confirm the widely held belief that addiction is not a medical illness and is therefore not significantly affected by medical interventions. On other hand, maybe the problem is instead related to current treatment strategies and outcome expectations, which view addiction as a curable, acute condition. Yet if addiction is more like diabetes than a broken leg, then the appropriate standards for treatment and outcome expectations would be those applied to other chronic illnesses and would focus on reduction rather than elimination of relapse, improved function, and quality of life.

In their concluding comments, the authors wrote that

similarities in heritability, course, and particularly response to treatment raise the question of why medical treatments are not seen as appropriate or effective when applied to alcohol and drug dependence. One possibility is the way drug dependence treatments have traditionally been delivered and evaluated.

Many drug dependence treatments are delivered in a manner that is more appropriate for acute care disorders. Many patients receive detoxification only. Others are admitted to specialty treatment programs, where the goal has been to rehabilitate and discharge them as one might rehabilitate a surgical patient following a joint replacement. Outcome evaluations are typically conducted 6 to 12 months following treatment discharge. The usual outcome evaluated is whether the patient has been continuously abstinent after leaving treatment.

Imagine this same strategy applied to the treatment of hypertension. Hypertensive patients would be admitted to a 28-day hypertension rehabilitation program, where they would receive group and individual counseling regarding behavioral control of diet, exercise, and lifestyle. Very few would be prescribed medications, since the prevailing insurance restrictions would discourage maintenance medications.[4] Patients completing the program would be discharged to community resources, typically without continued medical monitoring. An evaluation of these patients 6 to 12 months following discharge would count as successes only those who had remained continuously normotensive for the entire postdischarge period.

In this regard, it is interesting that relapse among patients with diabetes, hypertension, and asthma following cessation of treatment has been considered evidence of the effectiveness of those treatments and the need to retain patients in medical monitoring. In contrast, relapse to drug or alcohol use following discharge from addiction treatment has been considered evidence of treatment failure.

The paper is a passionate, elegant, and incontrovertible argument for why addiction treatment must focus on continuing care and disease management that involve behavioral interventions as well as relapse preventive medications, and that may require interventions and monitoring throughout the patient's lifespan. It explains why outcome expectations must reflect the chronic relapsing nature of the disease, rather than narrowly focusing on abstinence alone. It seems impossible for anyone involved in the treatment of patients with addictive disorders to read the paper without inferring that the entire treatment enterprise in this area needs to be fundamentally revamped. The paper is one of the most influential in the field of addiction in decades and has so far been cited over a thousand times by other scientists. These days I rarely review a research grant application that does not start out by stating that "addiction is a chronic, relapsing illness." By these measures, the paper has been as successful as a university professor can ever hope for when writing an academic piece. Devoting most of a chapter to reviewing its analysis and conclusions over a decade later may seem like a waste of time.

There is just one little problem. Despite everything, more than a decade later, very little has changed in the real world of addiction treatment. But before addressing the lack of progress, I must deal with another fundamental issue.

5

MAN OR MACHINE?

IN AN ENCOUNTER with a patient, every clinician is faced with a fundamental dilemma. Although present in all areas of medicine, this issue becomes most acute in psychiatry and behavioral health. In these fields, feelings, intentions, and decisions are at the core of the clinical disorders that bring patients to treatment. So the question cannot be avoided: should what happens in the patient's mind be viewed as yet another set of physiological processes, possible to register from the outside in an objective manner and to predictably manipulate with interventions such as drugs, similar to what we expect of blood pressure or serum glucose? Or are these inner processes inherently different from physiology, requiring that we view them as uniquely subjective, volitional processes of the mind? In other words, is the patient an agent expressing a unique free will or an object that follows deterministic[1] laws of nature? An inability to resolve this dilemma, or at least to find pragmatic ways of handling it, has been behind much of the tensions and feuds that have preoccupied psychiatry and related disciplines for more than a century. It has also diverted time and energy from developing, implementing, and providing better treatments for patients who need them. We cannot move on without addressing this issue.

In a way, every patient encounter is a mystery. After years of sobriety, the patient suddenly decides to drink again. Afterward, across the exam room, a fellow human is sharing that uniquely personal experience and the feelings, intentions, and decisions that went into it. I have no way of directly accessing the patient's mind. If I were required to provide scientific proof, I don't think I could even prove that the patient has a mind. But as I tune in, listen, and watch the expressions that accompany the account, I experience feelings of my own: sadness, anger, perhaps joy. Thoughts come to me about what may have happened. As is so often the case, something important about what is going on is embedded in the language used to describe it. I say that the patient's account strikes a chord or resonates with me. The image that comes to mind is that of two strings, on two separate instruments. One plays a tone, and the other, if properly tuned, is put in motion to play the same note, albeit with different overtones. In a clinical setting, this subtle process is critical. Developing an ability to tune in to uniquely subjective feelings of patients constitutes half the job skills required of any psychiatrist. Without this skill, it is hard to imagine how a clinician could ever connect with a patient suffering the intense sadness of a major depression, the irrational fears of an anxiety disorder, or the seemingly irresistible urges of addiction. Before patients will trust a doctor with what torments them and build the alliance necessary for the hard work of treatment to succeed, they want to know that the doctor has a sense of what they are experiencing and cares about it. Somehow, a process needs to take place that will ultimately enable one person to say "I feel your pain" and the other to trust that to be the case.

Stated differently, when experienced from the inside, the desires, fears, or intentions to act in a particular way have a peculiar subjective quality that is hard, if not impossible, for others to access. My desires and fears are mine. In fact, my desires and fears are *me*. The notion that other people, whom we can only observe from the outside, also have minds, feelings, and intentions is by no means self-evident. Who knows—maybe, unbeknown to me, I have been given Jim Carrey's role in a sequel to the 1998 movie *The Truman Show*. Maybe people around me are just playing roles scripted for them by a demonic movie director. Or maybe they are animated by a new technology from Pixar. It is surprisingly difficult to refute these obviously ridiculous notions, yet I take for granted that they are ridiculous. Instead I assume that people around me who speak, laugh, cry, or act do so because of feelings, intentions, and decisions similar to mine. That is because, like most healthy adult humans, I have developed what has come to be called a theory of mind.

This important concept, introduced by University of Pennsylvania primatologist David Premack and his colleague Guy Woodruff in 1978,[2] has been extensively studied since then. Human children begin to develop a theory of mind before the age of two, most likely by noticing similarities between themselves and others. The child feels happy and smiles. Mother is smiling too; perhaps she feels the same way? This way we grow up instinctively attributing to others feelings and intentions much like our own. But our own feelings, intentions, and decisions appear to us as primary, irreducible phenomena that ultimately cause our behavior. This appearance is unreflected, for the most part not explicitly articulated, and fully developed long before rationality or scientific training could allow us to probe its basis or limitations. Because this is the way we come to view ourselves, and because the theory of mind we apply to other people is based on attributing to them inner experiences similar to our own, we come to view other people in much the same way—as irreducible agents of their actions, actions carried out as a result of decisions that ultimately represent nothing less than the exercise of a free will. From that perspective maybe it is reasonable to hold that to stop using drugs, it is enough to "just say no."

And yet, at the same time, we know that patient histories are also quite predictable, in the best and clinically most useful sense of the word. If you tell me that you have been struggling with alcoholism for the past ten years and then take a drink, I can predict that on most occasions you will not stop at that one drink, even though you planned to. If you tell me that your father was an alcoholic, that you took your first drinks when you were fifteen, and that the friends with whom you were drinking fell asleep while you did not at all become impaired, I can predict that you run a high risk of developing alcohol problems in coming years. These are the kinds of predictions that medicine relies on for successful treatment, as well as successful prevention. Based on these kinds of predictions, we can intervene and say things such as "Let's practice behaviors that will help you avoid taking that first drink, and if you do practice enough to master them, we can predict that the probability of relapse will decrease." Or "Let's make sure you take a nalmefene tablet before going to a cocktail party, and we can predict a reduction in relapse risk." Perhaps more provocatively, "Stay on this antidepressant for four weeks, and we can predict that your existential despair will likely give way to an interest in repainting the garage or going to the movies with your wife." Viewed from this perspective, feelings, intentions, decisions, and actions certainly appear to be predictable, determined by factors that we can identify and sometimes influence—thus both objective entities and largely deterministic.

This is, of course, a very different perspective on feelings, intentions, and actions from that of empathically listening to a fellow human endowed with unique feelings and desires. Viewed this way, the mind content and behavior of people seem to follow laws of nature like any inanimate object. We may not yet have fully figured out the particular laws that are involved or possess the capacity to carry out the computations to predict outcomes in detail, but laws they are, nevertheless. This is likely the perspective of a trained scientist or an experienced clinician. It underlies the application of the medical model to brain diseases and brings with it all the power of modern medicine. British Nobel laureate Francis Crick provided an articulate account of this perspective in his book *An Astonishing Hypothesis* (1994):

> You, your joys and your sorrows, your memories and your ambitions, your sense of personal identity and free will, are in fact no more than the behavior of a vast assembly of nerve cells and their associated molecules. As Lewis Carroll's Alice might have phrased: "You're nothing but a pack of neurons." This hypothesis is so alien to the ideas of most people today that it can truly be called astonishing.

"Astonishing," as used here, is a nice British understatement. Unsettling, provocative, or infuriating are probably closer to the real meaning. In the abstract, people perhaps find this perspective on the mind somewhat less astonishing today than they did in 1994 when Crick put it forward. In everyday life the notion remains as foreign as ever. It brings with it the dilemma we are discussing, which paradoxically becomes worse as we become better at figuring out the laws of nature that govern brain function, improving our ability to make predictions and to influence outcomes in the domain of the mind. The crude and incorrect prediction that bloodletting would cure a mysterious fever probably did not offend many sensibilities, in part simply because it didn't work. But as science and medicine become capable of making powerful predictions about feelings, thoughts, and decisions, phenomena we have come to view as our innermost self for as long as we can remember, the challenge becomes unavoidable. The prediction that taking a medication will change one's outlook on whether life is worth living, or change one's willingness to stay sober, is just so much more provocative. It seems to reduce a human being, with all the woes and joys that flesh is heir to, to an object not much different from a complicated machine. From this perspective phenomena we view as our innermost self seem merely to be byproducts of sophisticated biological machinery.

Interestingly enough, people rarely have a problem with viewing the function of their cardiovascular systems as sophisticated machinery. Even if they don't know the laws of physiology that describe how this system delivers oxygen to tissues, they do not doubt that such laws exist and can be used to predictably influence heart rate or blood pressure with drugs. Bluntly stating that the same may apply to a person's mood or desire to stay sober will frequently just alienate that person. What? My secret desires, my deepest sorrows—does this insensitive jerk in a white coat really intend to reduce them to mere cogwheels in a machine and respond to them with a pill? Given that any progress in treatment relies on building an alliance, working together, and ultimately having patients take responsibility for their own treatment, alienating a patient like this is not a good start. Yet without interventions that have—at least statistically—predictable consequences, it is hard to see how a clinician might be able to help. What are we to do?

It is not all that hard. Stripped of ideological overtones, the simple fact is that both perspectives on the human mind outlined above are essential for a successful therapeutic relationship, and both are justified. What is critical is to realize when each of them is appropriate, and to develop an ability to shift between them. Every encounter with a patient must start with conveying a willingness to listen to and take in the subjective feelings of the patient. Some clinicians are easily moved and have a natural talent for establishing this connection. That is a true gift, but it also poses a distinct risk. We all like to do the things we are good at. If listening and using a well-developed ability for empathy is what a clinician is good at, that can end up being all that happens during a visit, and the next one, and the one after that. Although clearly valuable, being a good listener does not reach beyond what a sympathetic friend might be able to offer. A good working relationship starts by walking alongside the patient until a thread of trust has been woven. After that, however, a clinician needs to step back and apply the other perspective—objectively assessing behavior, brain function, and interventions that might predictably change mind contents and actions in the direction in which the patient has expressed a wish to walk. Or maybe the patient has not expressed any such wish; in such a case, as we will see in a subsequent chapter, there are psychological techniques to help him or her become more ready for the change that is necessary for improved health or perhaps even survival. Challenging though these perspective shifts are, they are one of the reasons I love clinical medicine, and psychiatry in particular. This marriage of science and humanism is hard to find in any other profession.

Although I find it impossible to apply the two perspectives to a person at the same time, I do not think that they are contradictory. At the core of every human mind are infinitely complex and subtle processes that we cannot access directly. Networks of neurons distributed through the brain come together in ensembles that fire in ever-changing patterns, but we can only infer their existence indirectly. The consequences of their workings can, however, obviously be viewed in many different ways. Each of these is as incomplete as it is indirect and can be likened to a window that allows only a limited view, from a certain restricted angle. Depending on which window we look through, things will look different. If the processes of the brain-mind are viewed through the window of a functional magnetic resonance imaging (fMRI) camera, they may look like colorful maps of activity.[3] Viewed through an electroencephalogram (EEG), they will appear as waveforms on paper. Viewed from the inside, they feel like—well, like me. But these perceptions and many others are simply different reflections of the same underlying processes that occur as infinitely complex neuronal ensembles fire in patterns that change on a millisecond to millisecond basis. None of the reflections is identical to the processes themselves; all are generated by those processes.[4] From this it follows that none of the perspectives on the mind outlined here is inherently right or wrong. Some are useful for some purposes, others for other purposes. This is not much different from saying that using a microscope would not be very helpful to perceive the beauty of a painting by my favorite painter, de Chirico. But the instrument would certainly be useful if I were charged with restoring the paint. So the antagonisms between different schools of thought in psychiatry strikes me as less an issue of being right than of choosing the right tool at the right time.

But before we choose that tool, we cannot escape one final philosophical issue. If subjective feelings, intentions, and decisions are indeed reflections of neuronal processes that can be objectively described and predicted, is there any room left for a free will? Or is it, against that background, not at all meaningful to have a dialogue with the patient about choices and their consequences? Maybe the only approach left to us once the neural processes are sufficiently well understood will be that of the police in Philip K. Dick's short story "The Minority Report" (1956): to predict undesirable behavior, and stop it before it happens?

This is one of the great unresolved questions of philosophy, and I clearly do not aspire to answer it. But I subscribe to a pragmatic approach to this problem that seems logically unassailable, which was proposed by the cognitive scientist and linguist Steven Pinker.[5] Pinker first notes that even if science were in principle able to fully describe and predict the human mind, it is unclear whether this would ever translate into an actual ability to predict behavior with a certainty sufficient to eliminate the perception of a free will. The brain may simply be too complex. But be that as it may, says Pinker, whether people have a free will or not, we all benefit from treating them— and being treated ourselves—as if they do. Pinker uses a drastic example. Let's say that person X is inclined to kill person Y. If X knows that he is viewed as being devoid of free will, he also knows that once he commits the murder, it will hardly be possible to hold him accountable. His behavior was deterministic—determined by his genes, the environment, or both. He had no choice. But if he knows that we believe all people have a freedom to choose and therefore intend to hold him accountable no matter what, the input to the calculations of his mind becomes different, and the crime is less likely to happen. Thus no matter what we think about the existence of free will and determinism, we all benefit from maintaining the notion that people can choose and take responsibility. Maybe this is an illusion. But, as it turns out, it is one that is both heartwarming and useful—a combination that is hard to argue with.

Having come this far, I hope you are ready to conclude that addiction is a brain disease, while agreeing that this view does nothing to diminish human dignity or to detract from the importance of listening to patients, applying empathy, and feeling their pain. With that, we should be ready to dive into the behavioral phenomena of addiction and the brain circuits that produce them.

6

HISTORIES, BRAINS,
AND BEHAVIORS

THE SMALL BAND of hunter-gatherers had been traversing the savannah for days, making good headway in the low morning light, resting in a patch of high grass through the hottest midday hours, and then moving on again, until the fall of darkness. A few days before, waving sticks and throwing stones, they had been able to chase off two hyenas and scavenge what remained of several antelope carcasses, left behind by some unknown predator. They had stayed at the site and feasted until no one could eat any more, and then used sharp stone tools to cut off the meat for drying and preserving. But for days now they had not been able to find water. At dusk the men sat and whispered while the women attended to the more and more lethargic children. The stream the band used to move toward during the dry season was nowhere to be found. In the end they had made their decision. The word traveled around the group, and once all the adults had nodded, the band started moving down the slope, toward the valley and the lake below.

The day turned to night, but this time they pressed on, some of them anxiously looking over their shoulders, others just quiet and determined. Hours later they saw the first moonlight reflected off the water. They pressed on until they reached the edge of the thick bush that bordered the last clearing separating them from the lake. They hunkered down at the edge of the bush, looking out for dangers in the night, pulled by opposing forces. The cool water lay before them. Looking down the gentle slope of the clearing, the thirsty travelers could almost feel a soothing, satisfying sensation on their cracked lips and dry tongues. But another force pulled them back. There was danger there, too. The men whispered to one another again. More than one of them had seen glittering eyes in the darkness or heard the sounds of struggle on a night like this, just before a member of the band was lost to an unseen hunter.

Some of the younger men were ready to take on any dangers. Others stayed still, as if frozen. In the end a scarred male who always seemed firmly planted in the ground raised his hand and spoke. It was true, he said, they had to have water. But leaving the bush and traversing the clearing at night was just too dangerous. They would wait until daylight, when the predators could be counted on to doze off in a lazy slumber. Only then would the band make its move. Some of the band members tried to object. One of the women pointed to her dry breasts and the baby she had put down on the ground, barely breathing now, with shallow, short breaths that almost didn't lift its chest. But the others knew the scarred man was right. They waited, biding their time, some drifting off into an uneasy slumber, others patiently staying awake, watching the stars move across the firmament. The baby gave up its last breath sometime before sunrise. Its mother cried quietly, rocking the little body back and forth while it lost its warmth in the cool predawn hour. Then, finally, heralded by a glorious aura, the ball of fire broke through the horizon, and sharp shadows started moving across the ground once again, marking the beginning of yet another day.

The band silently broke away from the bush and made their way down to the waterline. Once there, all but one of them laid face down, eagerly gulping down the clear lake water. The scarred man was the only one to wait just a bit longer, continuing to watch for dangers that might linger along the lakeside. Finally he too was convinced they were safe, at least for now. The baby had died, but the band had survived. And new babies would soon be born.

The complexity of the human brain is quite intimidating, even to those of us who have devoted our lives to exploring it. The estimated number of nerve cells, or neurons, in an adult brain was recently revised down but still stands at a mind-boggling eighty-five billion. Each of these cells has perhaps ten thousand connections, or synapses, that connect it to other neurons. Using different messengers, or transmitters, with an intensity that varies from millisecond to millisecond, these connections transmit information that is coded for most of its travel in much the same way as an FM radio transmitter codes its signal.[1] Over a longer period of time, the connections change in strength, based on prior experience and activity level. When the sparking of cells starts, a neuron comes together with others in a transiently formed ensemble that creates the brain's inner representation of a particular stimulus, a response, or some more abstract process that happens between those two. But the next moment, the same neuron will begin a dance with an entirely new set of partners, to represent something else. For now the question whether the workings of this machinery are in principle deterministic is hypothetical. Understanding what is going on and predicting how this complex machinery will respond to interventions are both challenges.

Scientists who try to understand the brain mechanisms of addiction take different approaches to these challenges. Some choose to study a model system that represents a tiny part of the big problem, but one that in return can be understood almost perfectly. For instance, some of the most advanced neuroscience research today applies a Nobel Prize–winning technique[2] to slices of a mouse or rat brain. While nerve cells in the slice are kept alive, minuscule electrodes allow the scientists to exactly measure the way communication between cells takes place. This kind of system allowed scientists to establish that exposure of the rat brain to a single dose of cocaine can change the strength of critical synaptic connections within what I soon will introduce as the "brain reward system," through a mechanism similar to that seen in memory formation.[3] Other investigators focus on problems at the other end of the spectrum. Studying the complex behaviors that the brain produces, they have, for instance, found that exposing cocaine or alcohol addicts to psychological stress makes them crave, and that the level of craving elicited in this manner predicts much of the risk for subsequent relapse.[4] Clearly the processes most obviously relevant for the clinical problems of addiction are also the most complex and hardest to measure in an objective and reliable manner. The most basic and well-defined experiments are, on the other hand, somewhat removed from the clinical problems of addiction. There is a whole world of intermediate levels in between.

It is not easy to know how to handle this dilemma. We hope that science will one day be able to connect these different levels of complexity, and that scientists will work on all of them. But for now the connections are just not there. Knowing that synaptic strength in a particular brain circuit changed because the patient took cocaine does not at present help me figure out how to manage cocaine addiction in the clinic. Until we have a more integrated understanding of how basic processes and complex behaviors are linked, we need to find a pragmatic level of simplification. On one hand, this simplified view should come close enough to the phenomena of drug seeking and relapse to help us make clinically useful predictions—for example, "If a medication can be found that will reduce the patient's reactivity to psychological stress by a certain amount, then that patient's risk of relapse over a certain period will be measurably reduced." On the other hand, this simplified view needs to be firmly grounded in what we currently know about basic molecular and cellular processes of the brain. It is not immediately obvious where this just-right amount of simplification lies. And we can hardly let this be decided by media reports of the latest hot story, which almost always are oversimplified, with a focus on the transmitter or gene *du jour*.

Useful guidance can, however, be obtained from a somewhat surprising source. A famous statement, put forward in a very different context, asserts: "Nothing in biology makes sense except in the light of evolution."[5] Immersed in the fast-paced, high-tech twenty-first-century world, it is easy to forget that our brains have been shaped by fundamental conditions of human existence that have remained unchanged in the hundred thousand or so years since we left our ancestral homes in Africa. Many of these fundamentals are captured in the brief episode from the history of our species recounted at the beginning of this chapter. As we are born, live, and die, our children and their children represent the only hope we have that life will continue, and so traits that help propagate the species evolve and become enriched in the population. While we live our individual lives, a peculiar excitement pulls us toward things desired, be they food, drink, or a prospective mate, or energizes the exploration of a novel place, where some of those desirable things might be found. Once the object of desire is reached, there is often—although certainly not always—pleasure.

But in a world full of dangers, unease, aversions, or outright fear constantly lurk as equally powerful forces, trying to steer us away from threats that otherwise might bring an end to the pursuit of our desires. There are, of course, many different kinds of fears and aversions, some of which we are born with. Faces, the most important communication device of our species at least until the smart phone was invented, are, for instance, detected by built-in brain hardware that needs only a few face-like features to flag them. And fearful faces, a sure sign that our peers have detected danger, reliably trigger fear responses in those who see them, without any learning being required. Other fears are learned. Perceptions that were once of little interest can become powerful triggers of fear if in the past they have been followed by distress. A third category, curiously enough, falls between the innate and learned fears: we are born with a preparedness to learn to fear them. It is, for instance, much easier to acquire a fear response to a snake-like object than to a rose-like one. Whether innate or learned, most of this happens quickly and beneath the level of consciousness. All of it is, of course, in the service of survival, without which no rewards are particularly meaningful. And beyond the acute fears there are other aversions, equally important for survival. In a pre-antibiotic era, disgust triggered by the smell of spoiled food was clearly a great help in avoiding death from food poisoning.

As the forces of reward seeking, on one hand, and fear and aversion, on the other, play tug-of-war within a person, a third category of processes arbitrates. Reason, much of which is concerned with planning for the future, helps the person trade off the rapid satisfaction that might come from pursuing desires against the need to avoid dangers. It also helps find a trade-off between the pursuit of immediate happiness, on one hand, and the achievement of greater but longer-term gains, on the other. For this, a whole set of new or improved tools are needed that are uniquely human; dogs don't have them, and chimps possess them only in a limited degree. For starters, there is a need for systems that can represent future, hypothetical states, a concept brilliantly captured in the famous expression "memory of the future."[6] Of course, multiple such "memories" need to be represented as possible alternatives, so perhaps "memory of multiple hypothetical futures" is a better, if less elegant, expression. Systems are then needed to assign values to these outcomes, also taking into account how far into the future they lie. Who knows? Putting off that dream vacation in order to purchase bonds that do not mature until a hundred years from now really does not make sense. The chances that I will still be around that far into the future are not very encouraging. But twenty-five years? Who knows? Choices, then, need to be made between the value-assigned outcomes, and these choices need to guide behavior, often by first suppressing what is going on already, and mustering the energy to switch gears.

In the end, it is the interplay of these forces and then some that allows humans to navigate the world in a way that is very different from that of all other species. The circuitries involved have different histories; some are ancient, others more recent. This history has shaped the relationship among the different processes, and their respective strength in modulating other circuits. It is also this history that suggests which behaviors might make sense to study in the laboratory using lower species such as mice and rats, and which may be sufficiently different in humans to make such studies difficult. And so a perspective on human behavior from the vantage point of our history as a species and the evolution of the brain is useful in learning how brain circuitry produces feelings, decisions, and behaviors that are at play every day of our lives. Yet it is that same circuitry and the same processes that make an addicted patient engage in the seemingly incomprehensible behaviors of addiction.

To put it bluntly, how can behaviors produced by brain circuitry that evolved to promote survival instead kill you?

It was late night, and I was getting frustrated. Months before, I had applied for a job I wasn't sure I really wanted—one that would mean a 50-mile commute each way and add to my already unbearable administrative duties. By now we had as a family decided we were instead moving back to Sweden, and I had just returned from a quick trip to finalize the details of the coming move. Funding was agreed on, space was selected, and the university had helped me get our girls signed up for a school that seemed quite good. After a night back home, I had packed a smaller suitcase and flown on to a conference in St. Louis when the phone call reached me: would I still like to give a job talk? Now I was back home once more, in my basement office, preparing for that talk. I sighed. At least this was an opportunity to do something scientists too rarely get to do, because we are constantly so busy generating data and writing empirical papers: sit back, read, and think.

The immediate problem was very specific. For the talk I could pick one or two particularly exciting datasets and use those to share my enthusiasm, point to research strategies I think hold promise in our field, and illustrate my vision for how science can address important problems of addiction. That kind of approach would be fun—there are few things I love more than real data. But it would necessarily leave out everything else. If I spent time talking about how genetics makes different people get different rewards from alcohol, people would likely think I subscribe to the view that rewarding properties of addictive drugs are what matters most for addiction. That leaves out a whole theme of how stress and negative emotions drive drug seeking, which I think is crucial, and to which I have devoted most of my own research efforts for many years. If instead I showed data on how anti-stress medications reduce drug seeking and taking, I would likely create the opposite impression. Showing a bit of each, I would have the worst talk possible: seemingly random fragments, joined by the arbitrary fact that they happened to be generated in my lab. Clearly I needed a framework within which to present selected data—a framework that would work for a one-hour talk to a diverse audience yet avoid offending some of the world leaders in addiction research who would also be listening.

I decided this was a time to try to convey my big-picture view of brains, behavior, and addictive drugs. Inspired, among other things, by a beautiful review article that was on my desk at the time,[7] I decided to fit the data I wanted to show into the three domains outlined above, represented by color-coded spheres. These spheres would represent the basic systems that execute brain functions I thought to be most important for addictive behaviors, and that could also be targeted for treatment, be it behavioral or pharmacological.

I needed to make three things clear: First, each of these systems can in turn obviously be broken down into ever more detailed subsystems, eventually all the way down to the individual synapse. Second, the boundaries of the main systems were to some extent arbitrarily drawn, so that parts of them could sometimes be viewed as participating in one or the other, depending perhaps on the circumstances. Third, a myriad of other processes were also important and not easy to fit into the three main systems but nevertheless relevant for what happens in addiction. Yet the three-sphere approach to brain circuits, behavior, and addiction actually turns out to be quite useful. And it does make perfect sense in the light of evolution.

7

THE PURSUIT OF HAPPINESS

O N JULY 4, 1776, the Second Continental Congress adopted Thomas Jefferson's view that the pursuit of happiness is one of the inalienable rights with which all men are endowed by their creator. The concept has been around longer than that, of course—for instance, as expressed here in a four-thousand-year-old Egyptian song:

> Let thy desire flourish,
> In order to let thy heart forget the beatifications for thee.
> Follow thy desire, as long as thou shalt live.
> Put myrrh upon thy head and clothing of fine linen upon thee,
> Being anointed with genuine marvels of the god's property.
> Set an increase to thy good things;
> Let not thy heart flag.
> Follow thy desire and thy good.
> Fulfill thy needs upon earth, after the command of thy heart,
> Until there come for thee that day of mourning.[1]

If, like Jefferson, you hold the truth to be self-evident that all people are endowed with the right to pursue happiness, you have probably just revealed yourself to be a somewhat secularized Westerner. A Buddhist

certainly would disagree, instead viewing the pursuit of happiness or pleasure as illusory while considering absence of pain and suffering, for oneself
as well as for others, to be a more worthy goal. But as we know, even within
the West and Christianity there have been, and remain, deep divisions
over the virtue of pursuing happiness in this life. Throughout the history
of humankind, our relationship to happiness, pleasure, or, to use the Greek
word, hedonism has been conflicted. That, as it happens, is for good reason.
We need to understand the attractions and dangers of seeking pleasure in
order to understand people's relationship to addictive drugs. Before we dive
into that material, here's a riddle to contemplate: find the word in Jefferson's
account that captures the most important aspect of these hedonic processes
as they relate to addictive disorders. Hint: it is not the word "happiness."
Keep thinking while we move on.

The concept of "brain reward systems" has since the early 1990s become
an integral part of the public parlance. The role of brain reward systems
and their neurotransmitters as mediators of pleasure is certainly part of the
conversation when discussing addictive drugs, and increasingly also when
someone has gambled away the family fortune, strayed from the marital
path, or become overweight. The concepts of brain reward systems and their
role in addiction have been so trivialized that I approach them with a certain apprehension. Yet they are fundamental for our discussion. To deal with
them, we first must follow them to their roots; to do so, we need to briefly
visit the roots of the reinforcement and reward concepts.

The fact that consequences of a behavior can reinforce that behavior is
classically modeled by an experimental animal that is able to obtain a food
pellet when it presses a lever under laboratory conditions.[2] This phenomenon
has been studied since the early days of behaviorism by scientists such as
Edward Lee Thorndyke, John B. Watson, and B. F. Skinner. To understand
the sea change that was to come, it is important to recognize a program-
matic principle of the behaviorist movement, as articulated by Watson and
his "methodological behaviorism." This school of thought went out of its way
to negate the relevance of any internal states for behaviors that could be reinforced by their outcomes. So we have to keep in mind that reinforcement,

in those days, was a purely descriptive, statistical term. Any consequence of a behavior that made that behavior happen again, with a higher frequency, was considered reinforcing. If approaching the pantry results in obtaining a cookie, the frequency with which I will venture to open the pantry can be expected to increase. But that is not supposed to say anything important or meaningful about how I feel when seeking out and consuming the cookies. Early in my medical training, this perspective on human behavior seemed to me so dry, sterile, and detached from the passions and pains of real patients I encountered that I shrugged it off and decided it had nothing to offer me. It took me almost two decades to reconsider that position, and then only partly.

It is generally held that the shift of focus from easily observable behaviors to internal mental processes can be attributed to the influential cognitive neuroscience movement.[3] In its broadest sense, cognition refers to all mental processes, but somehow cognitive neuroscience historically had little interest in motivation and emotion. Instead it focused on processes such as memory, attention, perception, action, and problem solving. Important though these are, it always seemed odd to me that so much more emphasis was placed on *how* people and animals executed mental processes than *why* they did so. From a clinical perspective, the latter seemed a lot more important. Today those divides have to some extent been bridged. Motivational and affective processes are increasingly recognized as the fundamental engines fueling other functions of the brain.

With that, it is clear that a major contribution to cracking open the black box of behaviorism was a chance finding made in 1954. That year Jim Olds was a postdoctoral fellow at McGill University in Montreal and seems to have had little interest in reinforcement or, for that matter, addiction. Instead he was using electrical stimulation of different sites in the rat brain to examine whether stimulating their activity could facilitate learning. In the course of that work, Olds made a classic discovery. In doing so, he showed the hallmark of the truly great scientist. Rather than writing off unexpected observations the way most people do, he paid attention to them and tried to understand what was going on. With the data themselves published in the best scientific journals,[4] the true excitement of the moment was perhaps best captured in an account by Olds many years later:

I applied a brief train of 60 cycle sine wave electrical current whenever the animal entered one corner of the enclosure. The animal did not stay away from that corner but rather came back quickly after a brief sortie which followed the first stimulation and came back even more quickly after a briefer sortie which followed the second stimulation. By the time the third electrical stimulus had been applied the animal seemed indubitably to be coming back for more.[5]

This suggested a logic that was then, and remains today, as attractively as it is deceptively simple. Some brain circuits, when activated by electrical stimulation, seemed to generate an internal state that was somehow pleasurable or otherwise desirable and therefore was pursued by the animal by returning to the place where that internal state had first been experienced.[6] Olds quickly realized the implications and took the observation one critical step further. He built a device in which the electric stimulus generator was connected to a pedal the rat could press, without any need for the experimenter to intervene. When the animal pressed the pedal, the generator was activated and delivered current to the intracranial electrode. Rats invariably went for the pedal and kept stimulating. It is difficult to account for this observation without accepting the notion that an internal state can be reinforcing. We may not be able to ask a rat whether it experiences pleasure or happiness while sending electric current into particular brain areas. But whatever the experience, the animal seems intent on vigorously pursuing it. Presumably the activation of some brain circuits generates internal states that can be said to reward and therefore reinforce behavior. With those observations, intracranial self-stimulation (ICSS) was born as a model to study endogenous brain reward circuits.

Many stories have been told about this famous experiment, but the fact is that the brain of the original rat was lost, so we are left to guess where exactly the electrode tip delivered the current in that first case. Anecdote has it that a student had done the surgery and had gravely misplaced the electrode, adding to the mystique of this serendipitous discovery. It is a good story, but extensive subsequent mapping has rendered it less important. Over time it became clear that stimulating a surprisingly large number of sites within the brain seemed rewarding, as determined by the ability of stimulation to maintain self-stimulation. Stimulation at most other sites did not influence self-stimulation behavior at all. Interestingly, when the electrode targeted yet a third set of sites, animals worked to *avoid* stimulation, hinting at the presence of circuitry that encoded aversive inner states.

Together these observations made Olds articulate the basic concept that the mammalian brain must be equipped with hard-wired reward systems, the activity of which motivates or reinforces behavior that results in approaching and obtaining "natural rewards," such as food, drink, or a mate. It was also clear that these systems could potentially be hijacked by processes that short-circuit the connection between engaging in the behavior and obtaining the natural reward. One way, shown by the original experiments, was to directly activate the reward circuitry using electric current. It was not far-fetched to dream up the idea that addictive drugs might accomplish something similar. In fact, although little noted at the time, there was another remarkable similarity between drug seeking and ICSS. Olds showed that a rat would be willing to traverse an electrified grid floor to access the pedal that delivered electric stimulation. More than half a century later, drug seeking despite adverse consequences remains a diagnostic criterion of addiction. In recent years this exact aspect has received renewed interest as an expression of compulsive drug seeking in trying to model addiction in experimental animals.[7]

It took almost three decades from these original discoveries until the critical neurocircuitry that supports ICSS and reward processing was outlined and it became widely accepted that Olds's original "hijacking" postulate might be largely correct.[8] One reason is perhaps that it first seemed as if too much of the brain was involved in reward. Another reason for the slow uptake was that at the time Olds published his discovery, the chemical anatomy of the brain was still in its infancy. It would be several years before the Swedish physician and pharmacologist Arvid Carlsson published his claim that dopamine was a neurotransmitter.[9] Few people believed Carlsson; it took until 2000 before he was rewarded for his discovery with the Nobel Prize. A third factor was that it took decades of perfecting the necessary neuroscience tools before the full picture emerged. One such tool was the development of a particular way to make dopamine neurons shine ("fluoresce") when exposed to ultraviolet light under the microscope.[10] Another was the development of early antipsychotic medications, which block one kind of dopamine receptors. Once those were discovered, it became possible to microinject them into tiny brain areas. That allowed scientists to map out places in the brain where these injections blocked a behavior. In this way it also became possible to show the role of the brain's own dopamine transmission in those places for that behavior.

Once all these pieces came together, a fairly consistent picture emerged. A major dopamine pathway of the brain starts out in the midbrain, or mesencephalon, in a tiny structure called the ventral tegmental area. In this structure, about half a million cells hug the midline from both sides,[11] about two-thirds of them containing dopamine. From here the dopamine cells send their nerve fibers to several different locations in the forebrain. One of those is the nucleus accumbens, the lower part of the larger basal ganglia system.[12] When this anatomy became well understood and the tools were in place, things came together. Animals would self-stimulate when the electrode tip was somewhere along the mesolimbic dopamine pathway from the ventral tegmental area to the nucleus accumbens. They would also do it with the electrode tip in places from which nerve fibers ran that in turn activated the mesolimbic dopamine pathway. Meanwhile, when tiny amounts of antipsychotics were injected into the nucleus accumbens to block dopamine receptors, animals stopped self-stimulating. And stimulants such as amphetamine and cocaine, which potently boost dopamine transmission in ways I will discuss in a later chapter, were also potently reinforcing when offered to a rat through an intravenous (IV) line. In fact, so strong was the reinforcing value that animals given unlimited access to the drug would lever press for IV cocaine at the expense of food, water, and sleep, to the point that 90 percent of them would die over the course of just one month.[13]

Self-administration as a measure of reward has obvious appeal, but it has also limitations. Most important, animals carry out this behavior with drug in their system. To make matters worse, the amounts of drug they are exposed to vary depending on the rates of self-administration. If the drug itself has an ability to influence behavior, it is easy to see that by looking at self-administration rates, we will be getting a mix of different effects. For instance, cocaine stimulates movement in general. Animals injected with cocaine run around more than before, and if they are placed in a box with levers, they will press those levers often, even if that action has no consequences. In contrast, heroin administration has a calming influence at higher doses. Animals curl up in a corner and become inactive. So comparing self-administration rates involves a mix of at least two different things: motivation, which is what we are interested in, and nonspecific motor effects, which we are not. A powerful approach to measuring drug reward in a drug-free state, called conditioned place preference (CPP), was therefore developed as a complement to self-administration studies.[14]

In a typical CPP experiment, a drug is repeatedly given to mice or other experimental animals in a distinctly recognizable environment, perhaps with striped walls and a grid floor. This is alternated with administering a saline solution in an environment that is clearly different—walls without a pattern, an even floor surface. After a few days of this, the animal is allowed to freely explore both environments, now connected with an open passage. No drug or saline injection is given. All the investigator is doing is watching how much time the animal spends on each side. This is much like asking the animal to reveal its preference for the drug memory. In this model, normal mice will show a high preference for an environment associated with drugs that are addictive, and also with natural rewards such food or sex. This has led scientists to conclude that conditioned place preference is a reasonable measure of reward. Recent work shows that it works in humans, too.[15] The most robust place preference is obtained with stimulants and opioids, but, similar to other addictive drugs, mice given alcohol show a preference for the environment associated with this drug.[16] Now, that rings a few bells. I could pull a patient chart almost at random and the pattern would be clear. Admission, detox, and discharge are followed by the patient gravitating back to an environment associated with drug use. This is one of the factors that ultimately set the scene for relapse, as will be discussed in a later chapter.

In the mid-1980s these various lines of research converged. A "psychomotor stimulant theory of addiction" was proposed, which built on the brain reward system theories of Olds and others but added to those the critical postulate that mesolimbic dopamine, through actions on the circuitry outlined by the self-stimulation studies, plays a critical role in the reinforcing properties of addictive drugs.[17] This theory seemed be proven beyond reasonable doubt when Urban Ungerstedt at the Karolinska Institute developed a technique to measure dopamine levels in the living brain while animals engaged in behavior. Using this technique, called brain microdialysis, Gaetano Di Chiara and his student Assunta Imperato in Cagliari, Sardinia, showed that most drugs abused by people potently increased levels of dopamine in the nucleus accumbens of rats.[18] A decade later Nora Volkow, currently director of the National Institute on Drug Abuse, carried out a series of human studies using positron emission tomography (PET). She could show that the subjective high people experienced after using cocaine or other stimulants was also associated with the boost these drugs give to dopamine neurotransmission in the nucleus accumbens.[19]

In the late 1990s it all seemed mostly settled, then. Brains had reward systems that use dopamine to drive approach behavior needed to obtain natural rewards. Addictive drugs were able to hijack people's lives because they hijack these endogenous reward systems and activate dopamine transmission directly. Because the activation they produce is so much higher than that triggered by natural rewards, and because they offer an opportunity to short-circuit the activation of reward systems without requiring the hard work needed for the normal rewards of life, drugs tend to win over natural rewards. For example, mating only doubles dopamine levels in the nucleus accumbens. Meanwhile, amphetamine increases them tenfold. No wonder amphetamine is more attractive!

There were variations on this general theme, mostly dealing with trying to sort out what dopamine was really doing. An important aspect seemed to be learning. Electric recordings in monkeys by Wolfram Schultz, then in Fribourg, Switzerland, indicated that dopamine provides a signal of something that became called reward prediction error:

Dopamine neurons are activated by rewarding events that are better than predicted, remain uninfluenced by events that are as good as predicted, and are depressed by events that are worse than predicted. By signaling rewards according to a prediction, dopamine responses have the . . . characteristics of a signal postulated by reinforcement learning theories.[20]

If this sounds too abstract, let's try again. Imagine you are strolling through the downtown of a city you recently moved to. You are not particularly familiar with the area. When you start feeling hungry, you don't know where to get good food. So you keep exploring for a while. Finally, in a side street, there is a little place that serves great falafels and is cheap, too. As you consume your meal, your mesolimbic dopamine neurons fire away. This was clearly better than expected. But a few months later, you know the city well. As you complete your shopping, you find yourself at the same food place almost without noticing it. Clearly you have by now learned what you need to do to get there. As you down the tasty falafel, those DA neurons of yours are largely silent. What would be the point of making any motivational noise? Things are just fine as they are. There is no need to drive your behavior in any other direction. In this context, the role of addictive drugs has sometimes been framed as being agents of pathological learning that somehow maintain their ability to activate dopamine neurotransmission over time.[21] This would clearly distinguish them from natural rewards, which over time become as good as expected, leading to a decline in their ability to activate the dopamine cells of the ventral tegmental area.

This was all fascinating, but as I was reading about these advances, I was toiling in an intense clinical service. And I could not figure out how any of it related to any patient I had ever had in treatment.

As modern times approached, the model outlined above increasingly became addiction science canon. It also became so engrained that the distinction between different drugs often was lost. What had been established for stimulants was automatically held to be true of other drugs, whether data to support that similarity were available or not.[22] Yet we have, for instance, long known that alcohol, the most commonly used addictive drug, has nowhere near the ability of cocaine or amphetamine to activate mesolimbic dopamine transmission. Microdialysis studies showed that self-administration of alcohol resulted in dopamine levels in the rat nucleus accumbens that were about double those at baseline, compared with the tenfold or so increase easily obtained in response to amphetamine. Meanwhile, several studies that no one wanted to remember had consistently shown that when dopamine cells were selectively killed using a toxin, rats happily continued to self-administer alcohol.[23] This was not exactly a ringing endorsement of a critical role for mesolimbic dopamine in alcohol addiction.

These findings clearly made it important to find out if alcohol does activate the classical brain reward circuitry in humans, similar to what had been shown for stimulants. The answer is actually a cautious "yes," but with an important twist, or several of them. In 2003 a study in eight Canadian men used a PET camera to show that drinking alcohol could indeed produce a measurable dopamine release in the nucleus accumbens. A few years later my late colleague Dan Hommer and his coworkers at the NIAAA used functional magnetic resonance imaging (fMRI) and also found that alcohol activated the nucleus accumbens. In their study, which for a serious scientific study got away with the unusually cute title "Why We Like to Drink," the degree of activation was also strongly correlated with the subjective feeling of intoxication.[24] Together these findings would seem to support an important role of classical brain reward circuitry in the pleasurable, reinforcing properties of alcohol, similar to stimulants. But it is critical to point out that both these studies were carried out in healthy, socially drinking participants. And even in this category of people, to get a robust response, the person should preferably be male[25] and have a particular genetic makeup.[26] When the same fMRI measures have been obtained from people with an increasing degree of alcohol problems, alcohol-induced nucleus accumbens activation has turned out to be progressively lower.[27] In severe, treatment-seeking alcoholics, there is simply nothing left of it, at least at levels of intoxication we can safely measure in the lab. That of course parallels patient reports that the high from alcohol declines over the years of being addicted. Yet these are also the patients that are the hardest to treat.

Systematic data like these are not available for other drugs, such as stimulants, but clinical experience suggests that this observation parallels what happens to people addicted to those drugs as well. Initially even a modest dose of amphetamine or cocaine will reliably produce a high in most people who try it. But for most patients with more advanced addiction to stimulants, the pleasurable effects wear off over the years and are largely gone by the time treatment is sought. That is why people keep pushing the doses ever higher. Yet despite the declining high in the late stages of addiction, the disease by then holds the patient in a much stronger grip than during the initial stages of experimental or recreational use.

So there is something strange going on here. We've said that the "pleasure signal" or, if you prefer, "reward prediction error signal" mediated by activation of brain reward systems is what allows addictive drugs to win the competition for a person's pursuits. If that is the case, how come addiction seems to be stronger in the late stages of the disease, when that signal has been weakened, compared with early on when it was fully active? Many physicians who work with addictive disorders find this problematic.

But maybe the dilemma is just apparent. Scientists studying natural rewards, such as food or drink, have for over half a century distinguished between two phases along the way to obtaining these goods. The motivation to seek out food when hungry is, intuitively, called appetitive. The affective consequences of achieving this goal are, in contrast, consummatory. Drawing further on the food parallel, it is not hard to design a thought experiment in which these two aspects of motivation can be disconnected from each other. Let's say that an evil thought experimenter fitted you with a cannula aimed for your nucleus accumbens, deprived you of food for a full day, and then let you out to roam the streets. Your appetitive incentive to seek out, say, the falafel place is clearly very high, and you pursue the search with vigor. But just as you find your goal and reach for your reward, a tiny dose of a medication that for a moment freezes the activity of your nucleus accumbens is deposited in your brain. The pleasure, or hedonic impact, of consuming the falafel suddenly turns out to be quite disappointing compared with your expectations. That, you may recall, is according to Schultz a great way to silence your dopamine neurons.

What if a mechanism existed by which the appetitive or incentive motivation to obtain a reward became progressively stronger, or "sensitized," while the hedonic impact of consuming the same reward decreased? People in whom this scenario had played out would more and more vigorously pursue their coveted reward, but the outcome would be increasingly disappointing. It is easy to see how this kind of process could lead to progressive escalation of both the efforts to obtain the reward and the amounts consumed. People would do almost anything in the hope of achieving the pleasure that was once there but now eludes them. Replace the falafel with alcohol and the description surely resembles advanced alcoholism.

The "incentive sensitization theory" of addiction put forward by Kent Berridge and Terry Robinson[28] is as sophisticated as it has been influential and is in principle able to reconcile the seemingly paradoxical observations that "rewarding" properties of addictive drugs tend to decline as people develop progressively more severe addictive disorders. In this conceptualization, there is no unitary brain reward system. Instead mesolimbic dopamine circuits promote incentive motivation that leads to drug *seeking*, and under the right—or rather wrong—conditions sensitizes over time as the individual uses drug. This motivation is famously called "wanting." In contrast, the pleasure from ultimately taking the drug is mediated by another mechanism, which may well decline over time. That hedonic impact is called "liking."

Remember the original meaning of the Greek root of "hedonic"? It means "sweet." Incidentally, sweet-tasting things make babies smile. It turns out that rats are no different, at least not once scientists learn to interpret their facial expressions. In a fascinating line of research, Kent Berridge has studied the neurobiology of these hedonic rat smiles. This research suggests that when hedonic hotspots in the brain are turned on by sweets, the pleasure or "liking" that follows "pursuit" or "wanting" is generated by its own brain machinery. These brain circuits are thought to be located in brain sites that overlap or are intertwined with those that produce pursuit, or "wanting," but the "liking" circuits seem to use different neurochemicals. The most important among those are endogenous morphine-like substances, or endorphins.[29] Endorphins may well be the oldest reward transmitters on the evolutionary block. They produce the pleasure that comes from the things that really matter in life, such as being held by your mother as a child or being stroked by your mate in adulthood.[30]

The discovery of endogenous opioids and their receptors has all the drama of the best detective stories. Beginning in the mid-1950s, it was speculated that the body may have a receptor for morphine, but at that time there was simply no way of showing it. Then, in the 1960s, chemists at the pharmaceutical company Sankyo tweaked the morphine molecule. In one of those tweaks, they ended up with something called naloxone, a medicine that was able to block all the actions of morphine, and that is still used in the clinic to treat heroin overdose. By tagging naloxone with a radioactive label that could be precisely measured, in 1973 Solomon Snyder at Johns Hopkins University and his graduate student Candace Pert were finally able to show the presence of opioid receptors in neural tissue.[31] Meanwhile, in Uppsala, Sweden, Lars Terenius and his colleagues found that the brain seemed to contain endogenous substances that bind to the same receptor as morphine.[32] And then Hans Kosterlitz, in Aberdeen, Scotland, together with his colleague John Hughes was able to fish out the first of these endogenous opioids, or endorphins.[33] It took only three years from the latter discovery, to 1978, before Snyder, Hughes, and Kosterlitz shared the Lasker Award, after the Nobel Prize the most prestigious award in medicine. It was widely expected that the Nobel Prize would follow, probably to be shared by Snyder, Kosterlitz, and Terenius. It didn't. In an unprecedented action, Candace Pert sued the Lasker jury for having left her out of the award. That was not the kind of publicity any prestigious award-granting institution wanted. The discovery of the endogenous opioids and their receptors became perhaps the greatest biomedical advance not to be rewarded with a Nobel Prize.[34]

The receptor that Snyder and Pert had found was labeled with the Greek letter μ (pronounced "mu"), simply as a shorthand for "morphine-receptor." As years went by, two other opioid receptors, kappa and delta, were also found, together with a lot of exciting science. For a while, based on pharmacological studies, scientists began to think there could be many more types of opioid receptors. But once molecular biology allowed genes to be cloned, it became clear that there are only three opioid receptor genes, from which the mu-, kappa-, and delta-opioid receptors are produced, respectively. After years of attempts, the delta-opioid receptor was the first of these to be cloned, in 1992, simultaneously and independently by Chris Evans of the University of California, Los Angeles, and Brigitte Kieffer in Strasbourg, France. The way cloning was done in those days, once you had one member of a gene family, it was easier to fish out other members. The cloning of the delta-receptor therefore gave the tools that soon allowed several groups to clone the mu-opioid receptor as well. As expected, it turned out to be central for the addictive properties of morphine and morphine-like drugs that I will discuss in a coming chapter. But in short, without the mu-receptor, mice would not self-administer heroin. And with the mu-receptor blocked, opiate addicts saw no value in taking the drug. They simply did not have the liking for it.

We will revisit if and how that knowledge can be used for treatment purposes, in the chapter on addiction medications. For now, let's just say that the mu-opioid receptors are in all the right places in the nervous system to produce the known effects of opioids. They are present at several levels along the pathway through which painful stimuli are funneled in from sensory detectors in the body and into the brain. This explains how activation of these receptors can dial down the flow of pain information into the brain and also decrease the "painfulness" value assigned to that information once it does reach the brain. The mu-opioid receptors are also present in the brain stem centers that pace breathing. And, most important for us, they are present at two critical stations along the mesolimbic dopamine pathway, which is thought to be critical for reward and approach behavior. Mu-opioid receptors are present at the beginning of this pathway, where the dopamine-producing nerve cells are located in the ventral tegmental area, and where mu-receptor activation turns on the dopamine neurons. And they are present at the site to which the dopamine cells send their nerve endings, the nucleus accumbens, a structure that opioid receptors can also activate directly.[35]

As we near the end of our discussion of "wanting" and "liking," what about the riddle at the beginning of this chapter? Returning to the incentive sensitization theory of addiction, we can perhaps now see that the key word in Jefferson's expression may not be "happiness" but rather "pursuit." To initiate the hard work of seeking drugs, the wanting machinery must be turned on. It is less critical how much the addict will like the drug once he or she actually gets it. To be honest, I am personally half fascinated, half skeptical whenever I read this theory. The incentive sensitization theory indeed has intellectual elegance to it when offering its explanation of how pursuit may intensify despite declining rewards. But it remains subject to vigorous debate in the addiction research community how important this theoretical framework is for the clinical realities of addiction. To me, the answer will be provided only once we find out whether the theory will help uncover any useful targets for successful addiction treatments. To date that has not been the case. But then again, the list of successful endeavors based on other approaches is quite short as well.

Meanwhile, there may be another set of reasons some people with addiction might continue to vigorously pursue drugs, despite the pleasure being all but gone: habit.

When dealing with drug seeking, we are, after all, talking about behaviors that happen in the form of coordinated movement programs. To obtain a reward, we must approach it. Approach should here be taken quite literally, meaning physically getting to the rewarding object and somehow grabbing it. In a novel environment, incentive motivation is great because it gets approach behaviors to flexibly adapt to changing needs and opportunities. But when motivated motor programs have successfully been executed often enough, it is no longer efficient to use the complicated motivational machinery to get them going. That is the reason frequently repeated behavior ultimately becomes solidified in stereotyped, almost automatically executed patterns.

In recent years the neurobiology of transitioning from goal-oriented, motivated behavior to actions that are habitual and automatic has become better understood. Although not all scientists agree, it has been suggested that dopamine transmission also has an important role for moving the drive to execute approach behavior from the nucleus accumbens to the part of the basal ganglia that lies just above it, the dorsal striatum.[36] This process has been proposed to play an important role for continued drug seeking and taking despite declining reward value and adverse consequences.[37]

This too may have parallels in clinical experience. It is certainly true that heavy, "habitual" smokers who have a pack of cigarettes readily available to them will tend to light up without giving it much thought, occasionally even showing surprise when the cigarette reaches their lips. It is also true that occasionally intravenous drug addicts will seek out needles and syringes, fill them with almost anything, and shoot up in a pattern that simply is not sensitive to the fact that they are unlikely to receive any pleasure from this action. But already in 2003 Robinson and Berridge made a powerful argument against habit formation as a major mechanism behind addictive disorders:

> Many aspects of addictive drug pursuit are flexible and not habitual. Human addicts face a situation different from rats that merely lever-press for drugs. We suspect that if animals were required to forage freely in a complex environment for drugs the picture seen in animal neuroscience might look more like the situation in human addiction, and automatic habit hypotheses would be less tempting. An addict who steals, another who scams, another who has the money and simply must negotiate a drug purchase—all face new and unique challenges with each new victim or negotiation. Instrumental ingenuity and variation are central to addictive drug pursuit in real life. When an addict's drugtaking ritual is interrupted, for example, by lack of available drugs, flexible and compulsive pursuit is brought to the fore. . . . The strongest . . . habit in the world does not explain the frantic behavior that ensues.[38]

Of course, a partial contribution from habit formation in some cases does not necessarily contradict a role for incentive sensitization or other mechanisms. Several of these could be at play simultaneously in the same individual during different stages of the addictive process, or in different individuals. I remain skeptical that habit formation would be a major cause behind continued drug use, mostly for the reasons advanced in the quote above. But in this case, as in the previous one, it is best to keep an open mind. We should let the utility of the model for developing successful treatments decide just how important it is.

Before leaving brain reward circuits, mesolimbic dopamine, endorphins, and the nucleus accumbens, I need to note a fundamental challenge facing much of the science I have just talked about. If dopamine activity in the nucleus accumbens drives the pursuit of drugs, is it increased or decreased activity of this system that makes a person vulnerable to drug use? I think it is fair to say that in the early days, most scientists made the assumption that the former would be the case. If taking a drug gave you more dopamine bang for your buck, you would be more at risk for finding drug use attractive. More recently, observations have been made that indicate just the opposite. For instance, most individuals who develop addictive disorders have lower numbers of a particular type of dopamine receptor in the nucleus accumbens. This is of course just a correlation and might in isolation mean nothing.

But other findings suggest that this "reward deficit syndrome" indeed might predispose individuals to escalation of drug use. Michael Nader and his team at Wake Forest University carried out one particularly elegant piece of work in support of this notion by using social manipulations in monkeys.[39] In these experiments, the scientists used a PET camera to measure the numbers of dopamine receptors. Socially isolated monkeys are miserable and have low receptor levels, but being in a group is not necessarily a picnic either. Some monkeys end up at the top of the social hierarchy, others at the bottom. It turns out that the stress of being a subordinate monkey, at the low end of the hierarchy, led to numbers of dopamine receptors that were as low as those in socially isolated monkeys. When the monkeys were then given access to intravenous cocaine, those with the low receptor numbers were the ones that self-administered the largest amounts of cocaine. This nicely ties in with a human study in which people with low numbers of dopamine receptors found the stimulant methylphenidate to be quite pleasurable, while those with high receptor numbers did not.[40] Maybe the reward deficit syndrome actually makes sense. Maybe an alternative to taking drugs for those who are at the bottom of society's ladder is to change the social order.

The reality is, unfortunately, likely to be a lot more messy. There is no question that things could play out according to the script of reward deficiency. But that does not mean that excessive rather than low activation of the same circuitry could not produce the same result. And beyond that, drug-seeking behavior is not determined by dopamine systems alone. The final go-no-go decision in pursuit of drugs is made through a vote between several subsystems of the brain, interacting with changing conditions of the environment and different properties of different drugs.

Frustrating though this may be, it is a great segue to the chapters that follow. There is, simply stated, a lot more to addiction than brain reward systems.

8

THE DARK SIDE OF ADDICTION

T WAS A slow Thursday afternoon. Perched in my office, I had finished up the paperwork earlier than expected and hoped to get to work on our latest research report. But a kind of weariness held me back. Instead I remained seated behind my desk, watching the gray daylight wane and turn into November dusk. The street below my window got busier and busier as the afternoon neared its end. There was a feeling of emptiness to what I was doing, one that has remained with me through the years and easily comes over me if I don't keep busy enough. It was never that way when I was a resident. Life could certainly be hell in those days, whether it was because one had to handle the admissions and discharges on a hectic ward or manage the flow of patients in the emergency room, but it never was boring. Preparing a report for the county's health care board sure was. I sighed and got my feet down from the desk. One of our doctors had just come by and said that the emergency room had a lot of work. It was two floors down by the elevator, then through an empty clinic corridor, to reach the back door to the emergency room. At first the resident working the shift did not look particularly happy to have the director come by and create a disruption. But once I looked in the ledger at the nursing station and quietly said I could take care of the next patient, there were no objections.

The patient has stuck with me to this very day. In a way, it is somewhat embarrassing that I peg my knowledge to individual patient experiences this way. After all, I have for more than twenty years passionately taught and promoted approaches to addiction treatment that are firmly based on systematically collected data, not the kind of anecdote that doctors or therapists frequently substitute for solid evidence. And yet this is probably the time to fess up. Without the archetypical patient who embodies the data, mechanisms, and ideas, I would not be able to conceptualize any of it. This is a quiet declaration of love: love of real clinical work, of the critical clinical observation. Love of that almost intangible perception that on its own may be entirely flawed and merely reflect the physician's preconceived notions but can also lead to systematic data collection and new knowledge.

The patient was a heroin addict with a scarf hiding injection marks on his neck. With that, I knew he had exhausted most of the veins we think of as places to inject. I could just imagine the rest. For a man, what is left at that stage is to inject into his genital veins. His general condition also reflected how far he had descended into misery, with dirty, disheveled clothes. There were pustules on his arms. A couple of them were open, and I realized that if I would ever be exposed to multiresistant staphylococci, this would be the day. He was shaking slightly even though we kept the exam rooms quite warm, and his nose was beginning to run with a thin discharge. Clearly he was beginning to go into opioid withdrawal. I got started on the somewhat obsessive ritual I always follow to obtain a history and do a physical. More often than one would think, this is what identifies signs or symptoms that are not obvious on a first look yet signal something that requires attention. Almost as important, the ritual itself helps establish a connection, a relationship that is a tool without which I frankly don't think any patient can or should be treated. At least not a patient that is awake.

Because I was just pitching in to help, there was no rush. No other patient was waiting for me. I took my time, and because of that I was struck by things we otherwise don't pay much attention to, things too philosophical to allow all the practical work to be done efficiently on a regular day at work.

The overarching question was simple. The extent of suffering experienced by my fellow human on the gurney was incomprehensible. He had already been hospitalized for overdoses several times. He was clearly well aware that next time could be the last if no one happened to be around to call an ambulance or do CPR. And if an overdose didn't kill him, sharing needles the way he did, he could be sure to contract HIV sooner or later. This was after the retroviral medications had transformed an HIV diagnosis from a death sentence to a chronic disease for most patients. But as my colleague who ran the HIV clinic used to point out, treatment works only if the patient has a place to put the medication bottles. Among homeless heroin addicts, death from AIDS remained a reality then and still does. I could go on, but the big question should be obvious. Because of the slow pace of the exam and the good rapport we were developing, I did ask. Why? Why would anyone in his right mind expose himself to this misery? The patient was, after all, a sensible person, someone with whom I could have a coherent, intelligent conversation. After all my years in addiction medicine, it remained a mystery to me how someone who seemed so reasonable could keep making choices that were so terrible, over and over again. Was the high from heroin really so overwhelming that it could just not be resisted? "Hell no. You know, Doc . . . here's the thing: when you start doing heroin, you really don't have to take it. But it is true, you just love what it does for you. Now, after all these years? I hate this shit, and it doesn't give me much of a high. It is just that somehow, it seems I can't be without it."

Despite the large number of scientific papers written on the topic, no one has in my experience captured what this chapter is about better than that heroin-addicted patient back in Stockholm.

"Give . . . wine unto those that be of heavy hearts."[1]

The notion that people take drugs to alleviate emotional pain rings intuitively true with patients, treatment providers, and many others. Often referred to as a "self-medication" view of addiction, this notion has had interesting ups and downs through the years. Following it through these cycles will allow us to better understand the flaws inherent in a naive, original version of the theory. It will also pave the way for a better informed and more useful modern interpretation.

Two men are usually credited with a version of the self-medication theory of addiction in the scientific sense of the word. They arrived at the concept from positions that were as different as the two men themselves seem to have been. Edward J. Khantzian, a psychoanalyst at Harvard Medical School, thought that many heroin-dependent patients had experienced difficulties with aggression, and that these difficulties seemed to precede their use of addictive drugs. According to Khantzian, these patients often reported that heroin gave them relief from dysphoric feelings. Based on these clinical observations, he concluded that a predisposition to become addicted to heroin resulted from problems with controlling and directing aggression.

In psychoanalytical terms, the inability to control aggression was seen as a result of "ego weakness" and was thought to pave the way for opioid use as a means of coping with poorly controlled aggressive drives. It did so, however, at the cost of producing physical dependence. Khantzian claimed that methadone maintenance could effectively manage heroin addiction not only because it controlled withdrawal symptoms and drug cravings, but also because it relieved the dysphoric feelings that resulted from unsuccessfully trying to cope with aggression. Based on this theory, in 1974 Khantzian and his colleagues published the original formulation of what would become the self-medication hypothesis of addiction. Over subsequent years, Khantzian went on to incorporate into his theory cocaine addiction, which he held to be a way of coping with depressed mood. He ultimately also included alcohol, which he thought offered closeness and affection to people who were otherwise not in touch with their feelings.[2] Overall, in this view, an addict's choice of drug was not a coincidence. Instead it reflected selecting a drug that offered opportunities to make up for failures to, as psychologists call it, "self-regulate."

A very different take on the self-medication theme originated with David F. Duncan of the Texas Research Institute of Mental Sciences. Duncan first noted that among individuals who engage in use of any addictive substance, only a minority go on to develop dependence. As discussed in a prior chapter, this observation was subsequently confirmed by the epidemiologist James Anthony at the Johns Hopkins School of Public Health. Duncan applied a rather straightforward behaviorist perspective to the use of addictive drugs but tried to sort out the different motivations that lead to recreational use or abuse, on one hand, and dependence, on the other. According to this perspective, use or abuse was driven by positive reinforcement, as also implied by studies showing that addictive drugs could activate and hijack brain reward systems. In dependence, however, drug use was instead thought to be driven by negative reinforcement.

Negative reinforcement is very different both from positive reinforcement and from punishment, with which it is often confused. To recap, positive reinforcement promotes behavior because an action is followed by desirable consequences. Punishment, of course, suppresses behavior by having it trigger aversive consequences. In contrast, negative reinforcement promotes a behavior because when that behavior is carried out, an unpleasant, aversive state is eliminated.[3] If my head hurts and I feel irritable arriving at work, I have a powerful incentive to press the buttons that deliver coffee from the espresso machine in our lab. Alleviating the aversive states associated with caffeine withdrawal by resuming drug intake is a classic case of negative reinforcement. Do note, at this point, an important distinction. Positive reinforcement is for the most part an equal opportunity motivator. In contrast, negative reinforcement practices affirmative action of sorts. It only affects someone who is already in an aversive state that can potentially be alleviated.

In any of these flavors, a self-medication view of addiction assumed that people who go on to develop addiction had suffered from preexisting conditions that involve negative emotional states, such as depressed mood, anxiety, or dysphoria. That is a testable hypothesis. Once it became the subject of systematic research rather than theorizing, the data simply did not seem to support it. In large epidemiological studies, addictive disorders such as alcoholism were much more strongly associated with antisocial personality disorder, a condition characterized by impulsivity and callousness, than with depression or anxiety. People with bipolar disorder, or what used to be called manic depressive illness, did clearly have a dramatically increased risk of addiction, but they are less than 1 percent of the population, so their increased vulnerability to addiction could not account for more than a small fraction of the 10–15 percent of people in the general population who develop addiction at some point in their lives. And people with bipolar disorder run their highest risk of drinking or using drugs when they are manic, not depressed.[4] Overall the bulk of addiction could simply not be attributed to conditions characterized by low mood or high anxiety.

Meanwhile clinical researchers found that use of drugs such as cocaine, heroin, or alcohol seemed to be producing anxiety and low mood, not the other way around. Negative emotions were most pronounced during acute withdrawal, which is when most patients are seen by doctors. If an alcohol-addicted patient managed to stay sober for somewhere between three and six weeks, the initially high levels of anxiety seemed to wear off in most cases. There was still a sizable fraction of people in whom these symptoms remained, but that fraction was no higher than that in the general population, where mood and anxiety disorders are quite common as well. Similar to the epidemiological data, these findings were not compatible with a view that conditions in which people suffer from negative emotions are a major predisposing factor for addiction. Instead it seemed that much of the association that clinicians and patients had observed had been the result of two things: transient withdrawal symptoms that were difficult to distinguish from independent anxiety or depression, and rates of genuine depression and anxiety that were no higher than in the general population.[5] To make studies even harder, there was frequently a distortion that easily happens when people are asked to report things in their past. This well-known "recall bias" is particularly strong when dealing with questions of addiction because of the stigma associated with substance use. Patients are simply more likely to report anxiety and depression as causes of substance use than the other way around.

By the time I was finishing my clinical psychiatry training in the mid-1990s, it had become widely accepted among practitioners of addiction medicine that talking about self-medication was mostly a distraction from maintaining sobriety or staying off drugs. General psychiatrists, patients, and the public of course continued to talk about self-medication. But then again, we knew that they were just not familiar with the data.

George Koob is quite a character. It took only a couple of weeks after I joined his lab in 1990 before he yelled at me in public. I wasn't doing rat surgeries the right way, meaning, of course, his way. To reinforce the message, pinned on the wall in his office was a cartoon, given to George by a former trainee, in which a Koob-like character said, "I'm always right!" surrounded by rats that were rolling with laughter. A couple of things made up for this style. First, George is one of the most brilliant neuroscientists I have ever met. Second, he is a great mentor who has continued to support his former trainees long after we have left his lab. The list of scientists he has successfully helped launch is long. When he received the Marlatt Mentorship Award from the Research Society on Alcoholism in 2012, it was after many generations of former trainees had come together in nominating him.

I had arrived at the high-energy microcosm of the Koob lab at the Scripps Research Institute in La Jolla, California, mostly by chance. My research love was stress, anxiety, and the brain systems that mediate these states. I had spent my graduate time studying a single neurotransmitter, recently discovered at the time. This work led to some important discoveries and revealed a previously unknown antistress system in the brain. It was a great training experience, but once I completed my degree, I wanted to broaden my views. I was also uncertain about my next steps, because even though I loved psychiatry, I enjoyed medicine just as much. Studying the role of stress in immunity seemed relevant to both and allowed me to put off the choice between the two specialties. I was therefore thrilled to land a prestigious Norman Cousins fellowship from UCLA to study stress and immunity.

Unfortunately, a few months after my arrival, things were not working out at the famous monkey laboratory I had joined. The lab was in decline, with its director, a wonderful psychiatrist, in ill health. I was simply not getting anything done. To make it worse, I found Los Angeles to be claustrophobic and depressing. As a last resort before throwing in the towel and returning home to do clinical work, I wrote George, on the off chance that he might have an opening on short notice. His response was characteristically Koobian. "I am booked with post-docs for the next five years. But do come and give a talk." I started in the lab only a few weeks later.

Two years prior to my arrival at Scripps, George and Floyd Bloom, neuroscience legend and department chair at the time, had jointly written a paper on the biological mechanisms of addiction that is still worthwhile reading.[6] It reviewed the accumulating data on the role of brain reward systems in addiction but also introduced the concept that prolonged drug use itself triggered long-term changes, or "adaptations," in brain function. It put forward the notion that these neuroadaptations fall into one of two broad categories. I have already touched on the first type, which affects the brain circuits that addictive drugs themselves primarily act on to produce their rewarding effects, such as the mesolimbic dopamine circuitry. Over time these systems become less responsive to drugs and also to natural rewards, creating, or perhaps exacerbating, a reward deficit syndrome. An example in this category would be the decrease in dopamine receptors discussed in the previous chapter. The authors called this type of change "within-systems adaptations," which I still find to be a helpful and intuitive term.

But with prolonged drug use, another category of adaptations, they claimed, would get under way in other brain systems. These would come online when addictive drugs caused excessive activity of brain reward circuitry and would attempt to counter the rewarding drug actions. The prediction was based on the idea that an organism attempts to maintain a reasonably neutral set point, or at least a range around a set point, for most of its important physiological functions, such as body temperature or blood pressure. Perhaps it did so for psychological processes as well? Perhaps prolonged and excessive euphoria simply is not a good idea? If, as discussed, pleasurable states and their anticipation once evolved to guide behavior in pursuit of things we need, having reward systems turned on and stay on in prolonged overdrive clearly defeats that purpose. Other brain systems would almost have to kick in and attempt to bring down mood to a normal range or else one would no longer be able to let good outcomes guide behavior. These normalizing forces, called between-systems adaptations because they bring online systems other than those directly activated by drugs, could be viewed as an attempt by the organism to keep emotions around a reasonable baseline or, in the words of scientists, maintain "affective homeostasis."

The notion of between-systems adaptations drew heavily on an influential psychological theory developed more than a decade earlier by the psychologist Richard Solomon, called the opponent process theory of motivation,[7] and generously credited by Koob and Bloom. Over the quarter century that has followed, Koob has progressively developed the concept of these opponent, counteracting processes. One important advance was the realization that the time course of these processes is critical. The "b-processes" that in Solomon's terms oppose the pleasurable drug actions frequently have a dynamic that is slower than that of the initial "a-process" of drug-induced high itself. When intoxication wears off and the influence of the a-process comes to an end, the opposing b-process is still active and pushes emotional balance below its original baseline. This activity results in the opposite of the pleasurable effects obtained during intoxication. In the absence of drug, there is now low mood and elevated anxiety. This is of course routinely experienced during alcohol or drug withdrawal. A bad hangover is, in miniature, an example of this "overshoot."

But there is a fundamental difference between a healthy brain and one that is addicted. In a healthy brain that does not shortly become exposed to drug again, the b-process will ultimately dissipate over time as well, and affective balance will be restored. Mood will return to a neutral level, anxiety will wear off, and sleep will normalize. The ability to guide behavior by its anticipated pleasurable outcomes will be restored. But this takes some time. If we take alcohol as an example, physical withdrawal peaks around three days and is gone by a week, but the negative emotions after a period of heavy use last quite a bit longer, often around a month, and longer in women than in men. If, in the meantime, the person attempts to improve the low mood by resuming drug use, he or she will be successful in the short term. But this will be at the cost of an even deeper suppression below the neutral baseline of emotionality once the drug effects come to an end. By now the intensity of the b-process has been further strengthened. What George Koob ultimately called "spiraling distress" is now under way, and in the absence of drug the patient is miserable. This misery can temporarily be alleviated by resumption of drug use, but each time, that is at the expense of further pushing along the process that makes the patient suffer even more in the absence of drug.

Finally, Koob adopted a concept from physiology, which outlines how organisms under challenge from changing demands of the environment can achieve stability by changing their original set point, but do so at the expense of increased wear and tear on their machinery.[8] In this he followed in the footsteps of one of the stress researchers we both may admire most, Bruce McEwen of Rockefeller University. Discussing a similar balance between the brain's stress and antistress systems, McEwen had picked up the "allostasis" concept from physiology. According to this notion, stability of emotions after prolonged stress or drug use can be maintained at a level different from that previously held, for instance, with more sensitivity to stress or lower spontaneous mood. Stability at this new level is achieved at a cost, called allostatic load. This is the wear and tear to the system that occurs when affective opponent processes are chronically turned on in a manner that is not supposed to happen in health, for instance the pleasure systems through chronic drug use, and the aversion systems in an attempt to counteract the chronic drug effects. This may all sound quite complicated, but think of it this way: affective balance is like a seesaw. The seesaw is balanced when children of approximately the same weight sit on each end. But it could just as well be balanced, in the same position, with a baby elephant on each end. Although the position of the seesaw would be the same in both situations, the strain on the teeter board, or the allostatic load it would be subjected to, would clearly be different in these two cases.[9]

These concepts were fascinating, but there was one problem in the early days of these advances. Despite the elegant theorizing, no one knew any specific biological process that would qualify as an opponent process whose activity could result in an allostatic shift of emotionality after prolonged drug use.

Rats and mice are just not great party animals. Most of them dislike the taste of alcohol and will not achieve blood alcohol levels beyond mild intoxication when offered free access to an alcohol solution. High levels of intoxication are an inherent element of alcohol addiction, so it is not clear how the low spontaneous consumption by a regular laboratory rat can be helpful for developing an understanding of alcoholism, let alone identifying medications to treat this condition. Medications that decrease the reward from alcohol can perhaps be expected to reduce motivation to drink whether an individual is dependent or not, so they may still show activity in the simple laboratory models. Later we will see that this is indeed the case with the approved medication naltrexone. But if it is true that the alcohol-addicted brain develops a set of adaptations that alter its function, and if these adaptations are important for maintaining addiction through negative reinforcement, then it is unclear how studying a normal, nonaddicted brain can be of much help. Yet that was the way the vast majority of alcohol research was carried out for a long time.

Research on other addictive drugs faces somewhat less of a challenge in this respect. Compared with alcohol, heroin and cocaine are so strongly reinforcing that animals will spontaneously self-administer them at levels clearly sufficient for intoxication. Ironically however, much of that advantage was lost for a long time because of the way research on these drugs was carried out. Self-administration was typically studied in short sessions of 30 to 120 minutes, during which animals quickly established stable rates of self-administration and could go on with daily sessions without many apparent adverse consequences for months.

We will revisit heroin and cocaine in a while, but alcohol offers the greatest challenge to achieving relevant levels of intoxication. As already discussed, it is less potent in its ability to activate brain reward systems. It is also taken orally, so there is a delay between intake and the psychotropic effects that weakens reinforcement. Also, similar to humans, animals that first encounter alcohol don't like its taste, which for starters at least further limits intake. There have been different attempts to address these challenges. One strategy has been to breed rats or mice that have a high preference for alcohol, just like dogs can be bred that are particularly keen to retrieve a bird or herd sheep. Alcohol-preferring rats and mice have successfully been bred in several laboratories and can be useful in searching for genetic factors that contribute to alcoholism risk.

But selectively bred animals don't tell us much about the biological events that occur as addiction develops in the brain. One approach that has been tried to get at this neuroadaptive process has been to let large numbers of rats have access to alcohol for a long time. After a year or so, about 10 percent of these animals begin to escalate their consumption in a way that appears similar to what happens among humans. That approach has a certain appeal, given that about the same percentage of humans given access to alcohol will develop problems. But even if the long-term-access model were to reflect processes similar to those that play out in people developing alcoholism, it is highly impractical as a research tool, and even more so for medications development. We need large numbers of animals to screen for new potential medications, and we need animals whose brains have been exposed to levels of alcohol similar to those experienced by patients. Both the level and the duration need to be sufficient to trigger the long-term changes in brain function that accompany the transition from occasional to heavy, addictive use.

Several ways have been developed to achieve adequate levels of intoxication that allow these neuroadaptations to be studied. Both my own lab and that of George Koob have largely settled on a method developed decades ago by a remarkable scientist and one of the pioneers of alcohol research, Dora "Dody" Goldstein. A graduate of the first class of female students admitted to Harvard Medical School and later professor of pharmacology at Stanford University, Goldstein invented a clever method to get mice physically dependent on alcohol. Alcohol was simply vaporized, and the vapor pumped into the enclosures in which the mice lived. This way they breathed alcohol vapor, which did not seem to bother them at all. They bypassed the limitations of taste aversion and easily became intoxicated. Goldstein was able to determine that a real withdrawal reaction occurred after intoxication was turned off, and she could study the detailed course of this reaction.[10] In Goldstein's experiments, the mice were made intoxicated for only three days, which was enough to produce physical dependence and withdrawal symptoms. Once symptoms had worn off, the mice were seemingly normal. But what if intoxication were maintained for a long time? Would there be consequences for things that matter for alcohol addiction?

Since 2000 a flurry of papers from several laboratories, including Koob's and my own, has established that this is indeed the case. Animals that have a long enough history of dependence develop a constellation of behavioral characteristics that seem to mimic core features of clinical alcohol addiction. First, they dramatically escalate their voluntary alcohol consumption when given a choice between alcohol and water. They are also willing to work harder for alcohol than animals without a history of dependence, indicating a higher motivation to obtain the drug. Their voluntary intake of alcohol that is offered to them remains escalated for many months, which is a large part of the life of a rat. Maybe this really is the rat or mouse version of the claim that "once an alcoholic, always an alcoholic."

Second, animals with a long history of physical dependence are more sensitive to stress. When tested a month or two after they have gone through physical withdrawal, they may on a superficial look not seem more anxious than are nondependent controls. One might in fact be tempted to think that they are back to normal, in parallel to what we found for alcoholic patients after a month or so of sobriety. But that is the static view. The picture changes dramatically if we apply a dynamic perspective and look at responses to stressors. At that point we will see something quite remarkable. A stressor of an intensity that does not at all bother nondependent animals will be enough to trigger a profound anxiety response in those that have a history of dependence. This seems to happen in people as well. When exposed to deeply disturbing images in a brain scanner, alcoholics activate brain circuits that process aversive stimuli to a much higher degree than do normal, nonaddicted people.

So it seems that both in rats and humans with alcohol dependence, a ticking bomb is present. It may not make much noise at rest but is set off when the individual is faced with a stressful challenge.[11] To patients, their families, and clinicians, this has a familiar ring. We have all experienced, over and over again, patient reports of how little things that once didn't bother them now totally throw them off.

This brings us to the final behavioral characteristic that develops after a history of dependence, which I think is important to highlight. To understand this characteristic, we first need to address the widespread notion that stress makes people drink and take drugs. A great deal of animal research has been carried out in an expectation that the same would be observed in rats and mice. But the notion that stress uniformly promotes alcohol intake is simply not true. Animals that do not have a history of dependence do not necessarily increase their alcohol or drug consumption when they experience stress. People who are not alcohol dependent don't crave alcohol or increase their consumption when stressed either.

But as a reflection of the all important neuroadaptations that are at the core of the addictive process, this changes dramatically if there is a history of dependence. Rats with such a history not only start out with higher alcohol consumption than those that have not been made dependent. When exposed to stress, they escalate their intake further. And what is perhaps most striking is that they remain at this high level even after stress exposure has come to an end. This, too, seems to have its parallel in humans. As I will discuss in more detail in a later chapter, people with alcohol or drug addiction experience profound cravings in response to stress, and stress is one of the major triggers of relapse in addicted patients. All this research seems to indicate that a history of dependence sets up a connection between stress and a motivation to consume alcohol that otherwise does not exist.

Although these mechanisms have been best worked out for alcohol, they seem to apply to other addictive drugs as well. For instance, it turns out that if laboratory rats are allowed to self-administer heroin for a long time every day instead of having the typical short access session, they will also escalate their self-administration rates over time, increase their motivation to work for the drug, experience an allostatic shift of their reward baseline, and turn up their sensitivity to stress.[12] Arming the ticking bomb of enhanced stress responses and negatively reinforced drug taking seem to be a phenomenon that happens with most drugs and affects both humans and lab animals. George Koob once gave it a catchy label: "the dark side of addiction." The question is, what neuroadaptations might be causing this shift in emotional state? If we could find out, we might be able to bring forward medications that can return this pathological state to a normal level. As we will see in the chapter on stress-induced relapse, science has identified some important brain systems that undergo dependence-induced neuroadaptations.

9

RASH ACTIONS

THE LITTLE GIRL'S birthday was less than a week away. Through the haze of cheap booze, her father dreaded the day. For months Carlos had not had a steady job. Instead he had been out on the street corner in Gaithersburg, where the jobless men gathered at six o'clock every morning, waiting for the beaten up trucks to come by and pick up a few of them for the odd job. He was drinking almost every day, but these were the times when there was still a lot of construction going on in the Washington, D.C., suburbs. The builders were not too picky, and somehow he managed to get work often enough to pay the bills. Then he got lucky. The foreman at one of the construction sites somehow came to like him, and there was going to be steady work for weeks to come, maybe longer. It was a long trip, and he didn't have a driver license or a car any more, but it was fine. He went first by bus, then by metro, then by another bus, relieved of the gnawing anxiety that there would not be any money that day. He still drank, but less now, and only in the evenings. And on the way home, as he stood up and held on to the handrail in the metro car, his lower back in pain after a long day of operating the cement mixer, he smiled. His daughter so badly wanted a new bike. She had outgrown the old one long ago and in the end had just stopped biking around with the other kids in the neighborhood, so that they would not tease her. Now, with the paycheck he was getting Friday, there was going to be enough to buy her a bike for her birthday. It wouldn't be new or fancy, just a used one from the Salvation Army store. But his little girl was not picky; she'd never had a chance to be. She would be happy. And so would he.

The week went by, and Carlos was ever so slowly and subtly being transformed back into his old self. During breaks, when previously he had walked aside and smoked his cigarette in silence, holding on to it with a shaking hand, he now stood with a group of the other construction workers. First he just quietly listened to the conversation, sometimes in English, more often in Spanish, nodding now and again, a little noticed bystander. But as the days went by, he made the occasional comment, sometimes asked a question. Over time, unnoticed, he became one of the crew. The conversation wasn't much: sports, money troubles, better jobs elsewhere, going back to a home that for almost all was somewhere else and seemed to be strangely transformed in memory with time, at once closer and farther away. He knew some of the men from other construction sites. They were all struggling, but most were good men. Most were married. What little money they made, they brought home, making sure their family made it through the day, week, or month, always hoping for the next day, week, or month to be better. Their wives worked long hours cleaning people's homes, or, if they were lucky, at the cash register in a retail store. Afterward they came home and made the money last longer by slowly cooking simple meats into stews that tasted of home or mending torn clothes so that the family could proudly go to church on Sunday and look the way you should in God's house. And then there were the children, most of whom spoke better English than their parents and struggled to understand whether their parents were there to take care of them or the other way around.

For Carlos, the mosaic of images from a life full of challenges had long been mercifully blurred by a cloud of drunkenness. Intoxication made everything vague and distant, softening the edges and soothing the unrest in his soul. Now, as he drank less and worked more, the clouds slowly started to part, and images broke through the haze. Some were so painful that he could not wait for them to fade away again: He is drunk. Marta yells at him, something about him being worthless and she would have been better off had she never married him. A rage beyond control rises up inside him, and he hits her, right in the face, with all his might. There is an awful thump, and before she falls, she goes completely silent, as if she were stunned by a Taser, unable to make a sound. And then, in his inner view, he turns around, and their little girl is curled up on the living room couch, as if she was trying to get as far away from them as possible, her eyes wide and black with terror, her mouth open, and tears forming in her eyes, before she screams out in desperation. But there are other images, too, some of which he tries to hold on to. Such as this one: It is a sunny Sunday in the fall, after church. They have borrowed Marta's sister's car to picnic at the lake. He and his daughter are throwing flat stones onto the lake. She is trying to make them bounce just the way he can, and this silly little skill for once makes him feel like she is looking up to him, the way a daughter should to a father. Meanwhile, Marta is putting food from the basket onto the picnic table and waving at them. These are the moments that make it all worthwhile.

When Friday comes, the paycheck is not quite as much as he had expected. Not much of a difference, but instead of satisfaction, there is a touch of disappointment. Something about new fees the county has put in place for the builders. The men are in no position to complain. And for Carlos, there is still enough to make this birthday celebration for his daughter count, maybe even make up for those birthdays he would rather forget. He has planned it all, with bike, cake, and balloons. But as he gets off the last bus and walks across the strip mall, music is streaming out of a bar. This is the place where he used to drink with his friends, long ago, before Marta, before their daughter, before the days of cheap wine or moonshine. He remembers sitting by the bar, being served rich, spicy food, watching a ballgame, downing beer and shots, dancing, and laughing so much that he could not understand how someone could have so much laughter inside him. Now, through the half-open door, someone calls out his name. It is a moment's work, and then he is sitting by the bar again, with men who may or may not know him, but who laugh just like he used to, until he, too, does.

For a while he tries to hold on to the plans he has made, but in vain. In a moment the mission he has been on for quite a while flickers for his inner eye and then goes out like a candle. Before it does, he thinks, "It is going to be all right. I still have until Sunday to fix this. I'll get the money somehow."

He doesn't.

What would you choose: a dollar today, or ten dollars a month from now? A hundred dollars today, or a thousand dollars a year from now? Easy, you may say, but there is in fact no answer that is always right. What is best depends on many factors. Some are of a universal nature—say, what a certain amount of money can buy. Others are unique to the individual making the choice. If you are terminally ill, receiving a thousand dollars a year from now may not be worth much. So it is clear that the utility, or "value," of the same outcome can differ depending on both the individual making the choice and the context in which the choice is made.[1]

There are other aspects, too, that complicate life. We may choose what seems to be "right" based on the expected value of an outcome, but what if it never materializes? It seems prudent to forsake a lower, immediate reward for one that is greater but will require us to wait. That is what we all try to teach our children. But when it comes to things that are more distant in the future, such as return on an investment with Lehman Brothers or payout from the GM retirement fund, there is clearly a risk that we will never get to enjoy the expected outcome. So in making their decisions, people also need to factor in risk and probabilities. If the person offering you money seems likely to skip town tomorrow, you are better off collecting what little you can up front instead of gambling on getting a higher return in an uncertain future. Whether we consciously identify them or not, we all struggle with these different factors that go into making reasonable decisions. What is most advantageous in each case depends on so many things: the effort required to achieve a desired outcome, its value, and the time and the many unknowns along the way to achieving it. To varying degrees, everyone will reduce, or "discount," the value of an outcome that lies in the future. Given all this, a certain degree of "temporal discounting" like that is reasonable. Too much, though, and you will never get the really valuable things in life.

Now, how about a drink today or a happy child fifteen years into the future? Addicts, it is often said, make bad choices. And for choices, people are held accountable to a higher degree than for desires, fears, or passions. Shooting a wife's lover is considered a crime of passion, widely viewed as an extenuating circumstance. Killing someone by driving drunk, in contrast, only aggravates culpability. This distinction contributes to the stigma of addiction and the often encountered view that an alcoholic with liver cirrhosis only has himself or herself to blame. Yet addicts are not alone in making choices with terrible consequences. Would I rather devour a steak for dinner and then crash on the couch in front of the TV, or eat broccoli and go out for a brisk walk? Go on vacation and pay for it with a credit card, or put more money into a retirement account? Drive an SUV today, or leave behind me a planet that is more livable for our children? Over the past decade or so, as both the importance and the complexity of people's decision making have become better appreciated, a whole new research field has emerged. Often labeled "neuroeconomics," this field has brought together an unusually diverse range of scientists, including economists, political scientists, neurobiologists, brain imagers, and addiction researchers. Plus, I suspect, a few people who would like to know how to set up a casino in the best way for people to lose money there. Decision making is key to whether people are able to cope with the ever-changing challenges of life and is at the core of the problem when they are unable to do so.

Interestingly, for most people, there is somehow a different flavor to the concept of decision making than to the idea of emotions. Decisions, perhaps in particular when made by the titans of Wall Street or investment bankers, somehow seem more cold-blooded and elevated, more "rational," than the hot emotions of desire and aversion. We even tend to use a brain word, "cerebral," to refer to this distinction. And yet from the perspective of brain science, it makes little if any sense to distinguish between processes that lead to plans and choices, on one hand, and those that produce desires and aversions, on the other. In fact these seemingly different processes are intimately linked. And all these functions must ultimately emanate from the activity of neuronal ensembles, firing away together at the right time and with the right pattern, be they distributed through one set of brain structures or another. Yet there has in our culture long been a history of what could be called a supremacism of rationality. As far back as Plato and

Aristotle, hot emotions have somehow been thought to be of a more lowly and primitive nature than the refined domain of reason.

That is because, in a way, they are more primitive. To understand this, there is a complication we have to handle, and handle with care. Yes, humans are in many ways similar to other animals. It is an undisputable fact that the brain circuitry handling the simpler of our desires and fears developed early in our evolutionary history and has since remained much unchanged, or, as the evolutionary biologist would say, "conserved." Because of that, the same brain areas—the nucleus accumbens, for instance—light up in a rat working for a tasty snack and in a human volunteer working for $5, or, for that matter, for a tasty snack.[2] The same goes for brain structures activated by anticipation of a modestly unpleasant electric shock, which will activate the amygdala and a network of structures connected to it in both cases. Yet it is equally true that we are also fundamentally different from other animals. Around the ancient machinery of motivation and emotion that we share with lower species, humans have wrapped a set of structures that have little or no precedent in evolution. Our frontal lobes are, relative to the size of our brains, larger than those of any other animal, except perhaps for the great apes. These frontal lobes are made up of characteristically human neocortex, which folds back on itself so that it can pack more nerve cells into the same space than would be possible had it been smooth like in other animals.

With the addition of these structures comes some unprecedented functionality. We no longer have to let our behavior be guided by decisions that are based on the value of immediate or near-immediate outcomes. Nor do we have to rely, for achieving longer-term objectives, on rigid behavioral programs that have proven beneficial through the evolutionary history of our species, the way a squirrel does when it collects nuts for the winter. We are the one species on the globe that has an ability to imagine a rather distant future, and ourselves in it. Because of that ability, we can flexibly plan for what may come. In fact, based on experience made during our own lifetime, or even that handed down to us from our ancestors in a book, we are able to imagine many alternative, hypothetical futures, assign value to them, and pursue complex behaviors that in the short term may require great effort for little reward but in the long term lead to an imagined future that seems to be a more desirable one. Because the world is a complex place, most of this has to happen quickly and intuitively, without reaching consciousness. An influential theory holds that imagining different "hypothetical futures" induces, in miniature, the body state we would experience if that particular outcome actually happened. That, in turn is monitored and evaluated by other parts of the frontal lobes, making us intuitively avoid a scenario associated with a body state, or "somatic marker," that is unpleasant and pursue it if the marker feels good. This may well be the true meaning of the expression "gut feeling," showing once again how much wisdom that can be embedded in language.[3]

To properly understand the relatively recently added functionality of being able to plan for the future, it is perhaps useful to remember that the evolutionary origin of our large frontal lobes is the part of the brain that moves our body, the motor cortex. This is the structure that forms a miniature human, or "homunculus," a map of the body famously mapped out through electric brain stimulation in the operating room by the neurosurgeon Wilder Penfield, founder of the Montreal Neurological Institute. The basic wiring diagram through which the motor cortex gets things moving, running through the spinal cord and out to the muscles, is reasonably similar in humans and other animals. But in front of the motor cortex, humans have continued to build more and more sophisticated computational machinery. By now we have grown our frontal lobes beyond recognition, wrapping them around the frontal poles like no other animals. So it is easy to forget that the "prefrontal cortex" is an extension of the motor cortex. But it is, and it guides behavior, which in the end is nothing but movement.

The difference, of course, is that the various areas that make up the prefrontal cortex do not move specific limbs. Instead they organize and guide all that movement, by doing many of the things needed for sensibly deciding on future objectives and planning for them. To get that job done, we need to represent in our minds future outcomes of behavior, assign value to them, and make decisions based on these assessments. We then need to monitor what actually happens, evaluate the difference between expected and actual outcomes, and update the valuation and decision functions once we have learned about those outcomes.[4] Other parts of the prefrontal cortex help coordinate these sophisticated processes and harbor[5] what is commonly referred to by the umbrella term "executive functions." These parts are in intimate communication with the valuation and decision circuitry and supervise its workings, making sure that attention is on the right topic at the right time, that the right information gets put into working memory when needed,[6] and that responses not aligned with longer-term objectives are properly inhibited.

Together, this is the machinery that makes it possible for some people to work hard on a meager stipend through years of graduate school, in the hope of one day becoming a well-regarded and perhaps even reasonably paid university professor. Or, more commonly, allows parents to give up on getting that fancy watch in order to buy their kids a present or put money into a college account. And it is this machinery that, had it functioned properly, would have helped Carlos make the decision to walk home after work instead of entering that bar, because the somatic marker associated with the latter scenario would have been unbearably repulsive. Except it didn't. Like many patients I've met, Carlos did not feel that sinking feeling, could not maintain attention on it, or somehow was unable to take it into account. That does not mean he was less devastated the next day, when the hypothetical future rapidly became a real "now." Neither does it mean he cared less about his daughter. It just meant that the machinery he would have needed to handle things was broken, through the double whammy of being born with ADHD that had never been treated and engaging in heavy alcohol use over many years.

A child is seated at a table on which a cake tin is placed. An experimenter removes the cake tin, which turns out to hide a pair of treats, for example, one marshmallow on one side and two on the other. The child is told that the experimenter will soon have to leave the room and come back after a while. To get the preferred treat, the child will have to wait until then. But the child is free to end the wait at any time simply by ringing a bell. In that case the experimenter will promptly return. The child will then get the less preferred treat at the expense of having to forgo the other one. So, in the most widely known version of this experiment, it is about choosing between getting one marshmallow now or two in fifteen minutes. Even in this simple task, where the value is clear, outcomes are certain, and the delay rather small, it takes some maturity to show the restraint needed to wait and earn the more desirable but delayed reward. In a series of classic experiments carried out at Stanford University in the early 1970s, Walter Mischel found that few preschool children were able to make it to ten minutes unless offered some distractions, and even then they didn't last a whole lot longer.[7]

Most adults, of course, can wait longer than that. The ability to guide decisions by outcomes that are distant in time is an important reflection of the frontal lobes doing their job. This and other frontal lobe functions are among the last to mature in an individual's development.[8] Adults also discount the value of outcomes that are distant in time, but to a much lesser extent than do adolescents or children. People do not reach their adult performance levels in this respect until they are around twenty-five, when their frontal lobes, to all parents' relief, finally achieve maturity. The same goes for other frontal lobe functions, such as a fully developed ability to suppress impulses or ability to avoid excessive risk.

Lack of maturity with regard to these functions can combine into a recipe for disastrously rash actions, in particular when highly attractive short-term rewards are present. Until such maturity is present, it takes quite a bit of adult supervision for those disasters to be avoided. As we know, because of poverty, broken-up families, parents who themselves are troubled, or just pure bad luck, that adult supervision is sometimes absent when it is most needed. That is when disasters often strike, in the form of fights, unprotected sex, teen pregnancy, drunk driving, drug use, or crime, in any combination. The actions involved often have terrible consequences not only for the individual carrying them out but also for others. Yet as a society we don't hold juveniles accountable for their rash actions to the same extent we do with adults. Even the present Supreme Court of the United States, not exactly a group of bleeding-heart liberals, has agreed that sentencing juveniles as adults would amount to "cruel and unusual punishment" because these individuals have a diminished, not yet fully developed ability to appreciate future consequences of their actions.[9]

It turns out that the capacity for delaying gratification, as well as other aspects of appreciating future consequences of actions, varies greatly between adults, too. In fact, although we all hopefully get better at it between the age of four and adulthood, the relative ability to resist temptations that are near in time turns out to be a rather stable trait for an individual. When the children in Mischel's studies were followed up, it turned out that their ability to delay gratification, as it had been determined at age four, predicted their ability to inhibit impulses later in life, both as adolescents and as adults. It also predicted their SAT scores, illustrating my father's creed that academic achievement is as much about patience and tenacity as it is about smarts. Recently these subjects, now in their mid-forties, were tested again. The behavioral differences were still there. Then a group of them had their brains scanned while being tested for the ability to inhibit responding when presented with an attractive stimulus. People who had been "high delayers" as children were still good at withholding these responses. When they did so, they activated parts of their prefrontal cortex. In contrast, "low delayers" did not activate prefrontal areas. Instead they activated their ventral striatum, the key node of brain reward circuitry whose activity promotes approach behaviors.[10]

The reason all this is so important is that being impulsive, as measured by excessive delay discounting, inability to suppress responses, and other measures, is one of the strongest risk factors for developing an addictive disorder. Yes, it is quite possible to be impulsive and nevertheless avoid getting in trouble. Growing up in a well-structured, supportive, and nurturing environment, a person who tends to be uninhibited will perhaps have a successful career as an actor or a snowboarder. Or maybe that person will boldly go where no one else has gone before in science. But under less ideal environmental conditions, or when not combined with special talents, impulsivity will often set an individual on a path to many problems, including drug and alcohol use. After all, the more advanced society becomes, the greater is the need for being attentive, carefully planning, and reliably exerting self-control to achieve success in most normal walks of life. Impulsive personality traits clearly interact in major ways with the environment but are also quite heritable, so more on this topic will follow in the next chapter. For now let's just say that, all else being equal, high impulsivity is associated with high addiction risk.[11]

How strong is the association? Pretty strong. Here is one clinically important observation that illustrates it: impulsivity is one of the defining features of ADHD. Sadly, but precisely the way it would be expected from this discussion, children with ADHD have about twice the risk of developing addiction compared with those without the condition. There is good news too, however. The elevated risk is for kids who do not receive treatment. In contrast, contrary to common fears and beliefs, those whose ADHD is adequately treated with stimulant medications have their risk of addiction reduced by half, down to levels that no longer differ from those in the general population.[12] Reducing impulsivity and improving attention seems to help in the real world. There is another piece of good news, too. It does not necessarily take medications to improve functions that are impaired in ADHD. In some ways, brain functions are like muscles. Practice strengthens them and makes perfect. So it should come as little surprise that practicing attention, response inhibition, and delaying gratification can improve those functions. By now there are computer games that allow ADHD kids to do just that: practice these things while having fun and being engaged. This has been shown to help with the problems of ADHD.[13] It remains to be shown if that kind of mental workout is also able to reduce addiction risk in these children when they grow up, but I would not be surprised if it does.

Clinicians have long known that patients with addictive disorders often seem to be more impulsive than people without them. But it has been hard to know what is causing what. Once someone has developed an addiction and seeks treatment, this becomes the proverbial chicken-and-egg problem. Most addictive drugs, including alcohol, increase impulsive behavior and risk taking by themselves, even when taken by healthy research volunteers in the laboratory. In addition, chronic drug use often results in damage to the frontal lobes, which in turn would be expected to further increase impulsivity.[14] How, then, can we figure out if the relationship between impulsivity and addiction is really causal in nature? Perhaps impulsivity has nothing to do with the risk of developing addiction after all? Perhaps its role is simply that it makes people sample the forbidden fruit more easily, and after that the addictive properties of the drug are all that matters? Or maybe the connection is even less direct. Maybe impulsive people, because they don't do as well in life as others, are more likely to become less well educated, poorer, and exposed to environments that are infested with drugs and crime? These issues have been much debated through the years. As is often the case, research in animal models can add a valuable perspective because it can distill complex questions like this and address them in less complex experimental models. Using that type of approach, research has provided support for the notion that impulsivity in itself is a major risk factor, not only for sampling addictive drugs but also for escalating drug use and transitioning from occasional drug use to addiction.

Almost twenty years ago, a team of researchers at the National Institutes of Health obtained some of the first animal data to support a link between impulsivity and addiction liability. Just like humans, our primate cousins the rhesus monkeys vary quite a bit in how much alcohol they will consume when given free access to an alcoholic drink. To people who work with them, they also seem to have very different personalities. Some are more aggressive, others less so. Some seem smarter than others. Could there also be consistent differences in impulsivity among them? To answer that question, one would have to come up with a method of measuring impulsivity in a way that makes sense for a monkey. In a series of experiments as brilliant as they were hilarious, that was just what Dee Higley, Markku Linnoila, and Steve Suomi did. Rhesus monkeys can all get around by jumping between trees, but different monkeys go about their transportation differently. Some play it safe, at the expense of not getting ahead very fast. Others take more risk and jump long distances. That allows them to move faster, but if they attempt jumps that are too long, there is a risk they will fall to the ground. That alone isn't really a good measure of impulsivity and risk taking. If they only try long leaps close to ground level, the worst that can happen is that they will have to climb back up in the tree again. But if they try a long jump high up and fail, they could really get hurt. It turns out that "long" for a rhesus means greater than 3 meters, and "high up" means more than 7 meters up in the air. Now find out for each monkey the number of these dangerous long jumps, divide by the total to account for the fact that different monkeys get around more or less, and we have a good, ecologically meaningful measure of impulsive behavior. Using that measure, it turns out that the most impulsive individuals in the rhesus troop are also the ones that will escalate their alcohol intake to the highest levels.[15]

Those data, or course, were obtained in the early days, when scientists did not pay much attention to the distinction between simply high intake of a drug and patterns of use that might be more relevant for addiction in humans. In more recent years, several laboratories have been successful in modeling "compulsive" drug taking, meaning that drug use is continued with high motivation, and even when it leads to adverse consequences. Based on those characteristics, David Belin, a French researcher working at Cambridge University's famous psychology department, assessed rats for individual differences in impulsivity and novelty seeking. These traits have both often been considered risk factors for addiction. Again, one has to ask, how could those behaviors be assessed in a way that makes sense for a rat? Novelty seeking is actually quite easy. This is all about how driven an individual is to explore a novel environment, so no matter what the species, it is probably enough if we can measure how vigorously that individual will explore novelty. But how about assessing impulsivity in a rat? Belin chose a test in which rats are trained to scan five holes and poke their nose into one of them when it is illuminated. If they do this, they get a food pellet. But after each time, they must hold back from responding for five seconds, until one of the holes is illuminated again. If the animal incorrectly pokes a hole that is not illuminated, it is punished by the reward being omitted, after which there will be a terribly frustrating five-second time-out. If the rat fails to wait for the light to come on and responds prematurely, it will be punished in the same manner. The premature responses provide a measure of impulsivity in the task. Using this model, Belin found that high novelty seekers among the rats initiated cocaine self-administration much faster than low novelty seekers. But once animals had initiated self-administration, the highly impulsive rats were the ones that made the transition to compulsive use.[16]

Interesting and elegant though this is, it still does not conclusively answer the question whether impulsivity is the cause rather than just a correlate of the addictive process. For all we know, both these behaviors could be independent consequences of some third, unknown factor. To conclusively determine causality, we would need some kind of intervention. Ideally, if impulsivity really *causes* addiction, we would like to see that suddenly losing key parts of the frontal lobes, together with the foresight they provide, should make a difference. Taking out the right parts of the frontal lobe should convert an individual previously not prone to addiction into one who does run a high risk of developing this condition. But this becomes a somewhat problematic proposition. I have discussed how key aspects of frontal lobe function are unique to humans, so animal experiments may have serious limitations. And an experiment that proposes to take out parts of the prefrontal cortex in humans may face some challenges in recruiting volunteers.

The famous case of Phineas Gage, and less renowned patients with accidental damage to their prefrontal cortex, seem, however, to support the argument. Gage was the railroad construction worker who survived after his skull was pierced in 1848. A 3-centimeter-thick iron rod passed through it as a projectile, sent on its way by a controlled explosion gone wrong during the building of a Vermont railroad. In the textbook account, this led to profound changes in Gage's behavior. A description of the consequences has made it into more than half of all undergraduate psychology textbooks. In this account, Gage turned from a responsible and trusted foreman at the railroad into a drifter showing a lack of foresight and judgment. What is less often discussed, but probably just as important, is that he also became, simply stated, a drunk.[17] Gage's case became a true celebrity in 1994. In a prequel to the *CSI* dramas of modern times, but in contrast to those carried out with an impeccable scientific quality, Gage's skull was borrowed from the Warren Anatomical Medical Museum at Harvard University and analyzed by the neurologist Antonio Damasio and his team, then at University of Iowa. The team applied modern imaging techniques to the skull and reconstructed the trajectory the iron rod must have taken. This allowed them to identify what parts of the brain the projectile had damaged. Between an entry point below the mandibular bone and an exit hole at the top of the skull, the damage appeared to have been in regions on the underbelly and the inside of the frontal lobes. The textbook account of Gage and his case has recently been called in question,[18] but the fact remains: in modern patients with brain lesions affecting the same areas as those the rod seems to have damaged in Gage, there is little impact on regular intellectual ability, such as that needed to solve math problems. Yet these individuals show a profound loss of judgment, foresight, and appropriate social behavior.

So the relationship between impulsivity and addiction is likely to go both ways. In the absence of protective family and societal factors, children who are impulsive run a much elevated risk for developing heavy drug use or addiction. Heavy chronic drug use, on the other hand, will make these individuals even more impulsive, in a truly vicious circle. By the time this dynamic has a person firmly in its grip, not even the happiness of a truly beloved child can successfully compete with the immediate attraction of a few drinks. This is not because the person is unable to do the math in theory. It is because when these real-life decisions are made, they are made in real time. And when that processing is carried out, the valuation, decision making, and behavioral inhibition machinery simply does not do the job it is supposed to do.

Decades of work in this field have convinced me that this is not a moral failing but rather a malfunction of sophisticated yet quite sensitive computational hardware. Some might disagree. Some might say, if all behavior can be reduced to the function or malfunction of brain machinery, then we are truly unable to make choices, there is no free will, and no one can be held accountable for their actions. And if that really is the case, then Adolf Hitler is no more culpable than the next person. I do not pretend to have an answer to this argument, and I agree that scientific understanding of how bad behavior happens should not be used to explain away individual responsibility. This dilemma has plagued philosophers for centuries. But I do know this: as he was admitted, after Marta had left him for their native Ecuador, taking their daughter with her, Carlos wished, at his core, that things had turned out different. After all these years working with patients who over and over fail to achieve what they seem to truly desire, I am convinced he wanted what most of us want. The difference is, the tools he had at his disposal let him down. Maybe if we can figure out how those tools work, we will be able to help people be touched by the better angels of their nature. That, I hope, is not too much to ask for.

10

TURNING ON A BRIGHT LIGHT

WHEN I FIRST met him, it was hard to imagine that for almost a decade, Peter had been chief of police in one of Sweden's major cities. After two weeks of having been listed as a missing person, he was found, disheveled and disoriented, in the rough streets behind the main train station in Denmark's capital, Copenhagen. When he was first picked up, I read in the Danish transfer notes, his clothes were dirty and torn, his body was bruised, and he was unable to identify himself. He was finally able to produce a name, a telephone number, and an address after a couple of nights at Copenhagen's large university hospital. By then he had been given IV fluids, had his wounds stitched and dressed, and been treated for severe alcohol withdrawal. His address, it turned out, was in a Swedish town just across the narrow strait that separates Denmark from Sweden. That town had an excellent hospital, so the plan was initially to transfer him there for whatever additional treatment that was needed. But the patient was not yet ready for anyone at home to find out about his predicament. He asked to be sent to any other hospital on the Swedish side that would take him. That was how he ended up on a gurney in front of me, in an exam room at St. Lars Psychiatric Hospital, a short drive south of his hometown.

It was my job as a resident to obtain the admission history. Early in my training, I had learned to follow a rigid routine when doing these interviews. Maybe it took a little longer to do it that way, but the reward was that in the end, I usually had a good picture, not only of the medical issues but also of the person. This time, however, as I was interviewing Peter for the intake chart, I could not figure out what kind of police officer this was. Then as now, I knew little about police work. But through a friend who was in law school, I knew that there were two very different career paths in the force. One was through the police academy, patrolling the streets, and perhaps making sergeant with time. The other was through law school, followed by a highly competitive police chief program that included basic police training and patrolling, all eight months of it, but recruited a very different type of person, with very different career prospects. The thing was, Peter didn't fit any of those categories. Over the next several days and a series of conversations that followed, it became clear why. My patient really was an unusual person. After a couple of years in the merchant marine following high school, he had first attended the police academy and started out as a regular cop on the beat. Along the way he had decided to obtain a law degree through night school, the first person ever to attend university in his family. He had graduated with top grades, despite working and attending school while also raising two sons together with his wife, an equally hardworking ambulance nurse. After that he became chief in record time.

Before he was discharged from the hospital, I had a chance to meet Peter's family, his deputy, the chair of the police board, and a few of his trusted colleagues. It was clear from talking to them that my patient was indeed an unusually capable person. Yet it was also clear that this was a person with rather severe alcohol addiction, so there were a few issues to sort through. Some were routine. Both the boys were still minors. Could we be sure that this was not a negligent or perhaps even abusive parent? As we all know, being a respected citizen is no guarantee against that. Was there a need to get child protection services involved? What about driving? Other questions, although less frequently encountered, were still standard. Sweden has highly restrictive gun laws, and with that, one of the lowest rates in the world of injuries caused by firearms. We would like to keep it that way. So a permit to own and carry a gun certainly had to be reevaluated in a person with an out-of-control addiction. But in the end, the job situation was the most unique and challenging issue. Could Peter really be trusted with commanding a sizable police force?

As we tried to gather information that would help with all these assessments, none of it really made sense. It was as if we were talking about two different people: the patient found behind the train station and the police chief. Everyone I met, superiors, colleagues, and subordinates alike, spoke of Peter as a hardworking, reliable, unusually conscientious person, equipped with excellent judgment. He never missed a day's work and was seen as a role model by his colleagues. Words that kept coming up were "unassuming," "caring," "a natural leader." In a job that frequently required difficult decisions, he seemed to have a rare gift for bringing people together, making sure everyone was heard, and then doing what needed to be done. And it seemed he somehow was able to do all that in a way that won respect even from those who disagreed. When I talked to his wife, she cried and spoke of him with unqualified love and trust. She seemed genuinely shocked by what had happened. His sons seemed to adore him and kept asking me if dad would get well soon.

What on earth was wrong?

In a way, it was actually quite simple. But let's start from the beginning. Peter grew up as the oldest son in a reasonably thriving blue-collar family, unremarkable except perhaps for their Pentecostal denomination. Because of his parents' religious affiliation, he did not encounter alcohol in the first eighteen years of his life. As far as he knew, no particular diseases ran in the family, and his two little brothers had done well in life. An average student and a better athlete, he went to sea, he said, because he had always wanted to experience the world beyond his small village on the plains of southern Sweden. Onboard it did not take long before he experienced alcohol for the first time. To his surprise, he found that it gave him an intense pleasure. He also discovered that he tolerated it better than most of his shipmates did. After a couple of years, however, he also noticed that the quantities he ended up drinking kept increasing, and he became concerned. He did not have any withdrawal symptoms, mind you. But even though he felt physically fine and ready for the next day's work, a lot of times he was unable to remember what had happened the night before.

An ugly street fight during which knives were flashed became a turning point. After that scare Peter went ashore, vowed never to drink again, and applied to the police academy. In secret he read every book on alcoholism and its management he could get his hands on. He learned the crucial habit of saying "no, thanks" when drinks were offered. In the end he decided to come out of the closet and joined a local Alcoholics Anonymous (AA) group. It was a step considered a bit unusual given his by then close to eight years of sobriety. It served him well, though. After a few years most of his friends and colleagues had forgotten his openly disclosed alcoholism or had come to regard it as something of the past. But along the way they also learned not to question his soft drinks at parties. And if they ever forgot, his quiet "no, thanks" did not require an explanation. "Ah, that's right. You are in AA."

And then there was an intense two-week course for police officials from all over the country. To celebrate its completion, the whole group took a short dinner cruise to Denmark. Onboard the ferry, good Danish food was served, together with cheap, tax-exempt alcohol. This was a group of people Peter did not know well, and they did not know him. When he was offered a drink, he told me, he could not in the moment find in his arsenal a response that would allow him to decline. After that first drink there was no going back and saying that, in fact, he did not drink. Of course, when we revisited this chain of events a couple of conversations later,[1] an additional reason emerged. That first drink had felt amazingly good. Over the years he had forgotten just *how* good. At the same time, it seemed entirely innocent. He was in control, among people he could trust. He took another one.

After that he did not stop for the better part of the two weeks it took before a Danish police patrol found him behind the railway station, beaten bloody.

Peter's story illustrates a fundamental tenet of addiction medicine. Remember, addiction is a chronic, relapsing illness. Anyone can stop taking drugs with relative ease. In fact, people with addiction do it all the time. In contrast, staying sober and eliminating or at least minimizing relapse in the long run is a tremendous challenge. To successfully treat addiction, we need to understand what triggers relapse, what mechanisms are involved when it happens, and how we can intervene in those mechanisms to prevent relapse. So here comes critical lesson number one: reexposing the brain of an addicted person to a small amount of drug is one of the most powerful triggers for relapse. The phenomenon, called priming, is simply striking in countless clinical histories. As the Big Book of Alcoholics Anonymous wisely teaches, "the real alcoholic does not have a defense against the first drink."

The priming phenomenon has in recent years been possible to replicate in the laboratory. Doing so has allowed scientists to map out brain circuitry and molecular signals that are involved when a priming dose of drug leads someone to resume drug seeking and taking. This is a good place to introduce what has almost become a standard model of relapse in basic science laboratories around the world. Introducing this model will nicely show how basic and clinical science are coming together in the field of addiction research.

The basic principle of the relapse model is first to train an animal so that it learns to self-administer an addictive drug. This, as already discussed, is typically done by allowing it to press a lever that delivers the drug. But in the relapse model, once the animal has learned to lever press at stable rates, drug delivery stops. Pressing the lever no longer has any foreseeable consequences. If daily sessions are run under these new conditions, animals will press the lever less and less, until the behavior is almost entirely "extinguished." Extinction usually takes a week or two, but in the end, the rates of lever pressing decline to what they were before the drug was offered. One might be tempted to think that this is a boring, passive process of forgetting. Maybe the memory of self-administration has just faded away? It hasn't. Under the surface, the old memory trace is still there, dormant, but ready to kick in on a moment's notice. One powerful way to reveal it is to give the animal a small, priming dose of drug. The animal will then run back to the lever that used to deliver the drug and resume pressing, at rates similar to those that were observed when drug was still available. This model is commonly called reinstatement of drug seeking. Originally developed in the late 1980s by Jane Stewart of Concordia University in Montreal and her student at the time, Harriet de Wit,[2] it has perhaps most successfully been used to understand relapse by the research group of another Stewart trainee. In 2006 Yavin Shaham of the National Institute on Drug Abuse received the Jacob P. Waletzky Memorial Award from the Society for Neuroscience for these contributions.[3]

Reinstatement occurs in response to priming doses of drug, and also, as I will discuss in coming chapters, in response to other stimuli known to trigger relapse in addicted patients.[4] It seems that once drug seeking and self-administration have become established, the brain processes that underlie them never fully go away. In that sense there may be a degree of truth to the statement "once an addict, always an addict." This is a disturbing contention, but it does seem to be supported by the laboratory data. For instance, initial training to establish self-administration takes a while and requires in the case of alcohol at least some clever manipulations before stable rates of lever pressing are achieved. Yet after extinction, stimuli that trigger relapse in patients make experimental animals resume pressing the lever that used to deliver the drug with no delay. A memory trace of the behavior seems to be stored somewhere, ready to be reactivated. In fact, we can reveal that stored trace. If we inactivate a particular part of the frontal lobe, lever pressing in pursuit of drug will reemerge in the absence of any meaningful trigger.[5] Whatever memory trace or behavioral program that was established for self-administration to occur must have remained in place, albeit suppressed and therefore inactive. Rather than representing a passive fading away and reverting to the original, drug-naïve state, extinction seems to have been an active process that superimposed new learning onto previously learned behavior of self-administration and suppressed it.[6]

Ability to block relapse induced by priming is of critical clinical importance. I will discuss addiction medications in considerable detail in coming chapters. But I have already mentioned Chuck O'Brien, who together with his team discovered naltrexone as a treatment for alcoholism in the early 1990s, a discovery for which he received the Jellinek Memorial Award in 2012. The now classical study from 1992 that first established the efficacy of naltrexone[7] might never have become the groundbreaking discovery it turned into had Chuck not as a clinician understood the relationship between priming and relapse. To appreciate this, one has to know some things about choices facing an investigator when designing a study to evaluate a new alcoholism treatment. One of the most important choices is what outcome to use in determining whether the medication works. Although this may sound trivial, it isn't. A typical research study goes on for three or perhaps six months. In contrast, most of the important things we would like to improve in the lives of people with addictive disorders, such as medical complications and disruption of family life, happen on a time scale of years to decades. So in designing a study, we have to pick something that we can measure in the limited timeframe available to us, but that at the same time can tell us something about the longer-term outcomes in real life. With alcohol, then as now, total abstinence was the only treatment outcome thought to be relevant. Importantly, that was for a long time also the position of the U.S. Food and Drug Administration. Yet it is clear that relapse to heavy drinking is what causes harm, not consuming the occasional drink or two.

Now, under most clinical conditions, that distinction does not make a whole lot of a difference in a patient with alcoholism, simply because the latter most of the time will lead to the former. So I hasten to say that I do not advise anyone who has developed alcoholism to attempt to achieve controlled drinking on his or her own.[8] But what if there were a medication that prevented the progression from a priming dose of alcohol, or a "slip," to relapse to heavy drinking? Initial clinical observations seemed to indicate that naltrexone might do just that. So that was what the University of Pennsylvania team decided to test in a controlled study. But the effect of naltrexone would have escaped discovery had the study team chosen the more conventional outcome measure—ability to produce abstinence.

As an aside, two decades later, a medication that is a cousin of naltrexone, nalmefene, has just demonstrated its ability to reduce relapse to heavy drinking. Based on these data, the European Medicines Agency has now approved nalmefene for treatment. What is noteworthy is the intended use. The company that markets nalmefene sought approval for "targeted use," which means specifically to block the progression from light, controlled drinking to relapse and heavy consumption. When patients know that they might soon find themselves in situations of increased risk for priming-induced relapse, such as onboard a ferryboat to Copenhagen, they will soon be able to use nalmefene as a pretreatment. Had Peter had access to this medication, he might have avoided the near-death experience that led him to the streets behind Copenhagen's station.

Fortunately, Peter seemed to do well even in the absence of this tool. For the close to five years that I continued, on and off, to work at the psychiatric hospital and kept a mailbox there, he sent me Christmas cards. It was in one of those he mentioned a conversation with his aging father. Only in the course of that conversation did he learn that, as a young man, his father had almost gone under from alcoholism. He had turned to the Pentecostal Church and absolutism literally to be saved.

Peter was atypical in many ways. The ability to stay free from relapse for so many years is in itself unusual in more severe cases of alcoholism, those I call "clinical," or treatment seeking. The resources he had available to him, such as a great job, a wonderful family, character strength, social skills, and everything else that had made Peter so successful for all but two weeks of the time I got a glimpse of his life are, unfortunately, not typical of patients who seek treatment for addictive disorders. Perhaps most important, Peter had an unusual ability for self-reflection. And yet it was a very different patient who brought home to me what this whole thing with priming is about at some fundamental human level.

Lars was homeless, was severely alcohol addicted, and rarely managed to stay sober for more than a week. When I met him, in a visit that created little more than a snapshot along a long, drawn-out process of ever-worsening health, dental status, and social situation, I was still young and naïve. I looked in his chart, saw the lab values that indicated ongoing liver inflammation, and informed him about the dangers to his liver in my most serious doctor voice. He nodded but didn't show much else of a reaction. It was clear that I was sharing old news. I didn't get it. He knew his liver was well on its way to cirrhosis. This is a condition that in the absence of a liver transplant invariably leads to a painful death, or rather one that involves literally itching to death, which is worse. And yet he not only drank but drank enormous quantities of moonshine.

I tried to challenge him to explain how this could happen. He shook his head. "You don't understand, Doc. I just drink a beer. After that, a bright light is on in my head. Once that happens, I am helpless." It is true, I did not understand. I had never in my life experienced anything that powerful. But his drinking buddies did understand, all right. These were guys among whom money wasn't exactly plentiful. Buying each other drinks wasn't common. My patient never had any money at all, so it was first a mystery to me how, time after time, he could find himself at a restaurant table, drinking beer that even in those days didn't cost less than $10 a pint with all those Swedish taxes. More in-depth questioning revealed the secret. My patient may not have had any money, but he did have a contact where cheap moonshine could be bought. He wouldn't give up that contact to anyone, for fear of losing it. The bootlegger didn't care much for visits from people he did not know, who might be plainclothes police officers. But my patient's drinking buddies had figured out that if they bought him a beer or two, just enough to turn on that bright light inside his head, nothing could stop him from seeking out his supplier and coming back with a large plastic container of booze. The return on investment was clearly worth it. They were happy to pay, every time.

It is clear that these guys knew a lot more about priming-induced reinstatement than I did in those days. They were effectively able to use their empirical knowledge of the phenomenon to achieve their objectives. This was almost thirty years ago, in 1985. Incidentally, it preceded the publication of the seminal animal model papers on priming-induced reinstatement by several years. I have been working hard to catch up ever since, and so has much of the field.

11

GETTING THE CUE

As I WALK down the street in downtown Bethesda on a warm Thursday evening, an inexplicable, intense urge to smoke hits me out of the blue. This is quite strange. I have not smoked more than the occasional cigarette in the close to twenty years since I met my wife. Yet in an instant, it is all upon me. I have the intense feeling that something is missing. My mouth is wetting in anticipation of the taste of a smoke, and I'm almost feeling a miniature preview of that taste, out of thin air. Similarly, my head is going just a tiny bit dizzy, the way it would do a lot more were I really to inhale some smoke. Yes, this is strange indeed. Why would this long forgotten set of feelings be upon me now, after a busy day at work, heading for the restaurant I favor for an occasional happy hour with colleagues from the lab? It is only a moment later that the answer becomes clear to me. As I turn the corner, standing on the sidewalk are two men, engaged in a conversation, each drawing heavily on a cigarette. I realize now that a faint smell of smoke must have hit me before I saw them. That, in itself, is not at all strange. The strange thing is that my first percept was not "there is a smell of cigarette smoke here." The first percept was "I need a smoke."

Here is a less benign version of the same thing. In 1977, when much of addiction psychiatry was still busy debating what kind of unresolved intrapsychic conflicts caused and maintained addiction and what kind of psychoanalytic approach might be appropriate to treat it, Chuck O'Brien brought heroin addicts into the lab at the University of Pennsylvania. Over several weeks he and his colleagues used an experimental procedure to let subjects learn to associate two simple stimuli—a 700 Hz tone and an odor—with the experience of heroin withdrawal that the researchers induced using a medication.[1] At the end of the experimental series, it was sufficient to present the tone and the odor alone, without any drug injection, for subjects to experience all the signs of withdrawal. These signs included the well-known objective symptoms, such as an increased rate of breathing, decreased skin temperature, and changes in pupil diameter. But subjects also reported experiencing the subjective feelings of withdrawal, which include an urge to take heroin. Clearly stimuli that were initially completely unrelated to any drug experience had by now somehow taken on a role as triggers for an entire coordinated program of responses, one that included unpleasant bodily as well as psychological elements. These responses were of the same nature that out on the street would provide a powerful incentive to resume drug seeking and taking.

I recall Chuck telling us a rather sad story related to this shortly after I first met him, one that brings these experimental findings out of the lab and into the real world of addiction better than most things I have since read in research papers. Chuck told us of giving a lecture for a group of physicians. As he had explained the objectives, the experimental design, and finally the results of the study described above, he said, a person in the audience, seated in the front row, seemed more and more distressed. As the lecture unfolded, the listener became increasingly tense and pale and started fidgeting with his hands. As often is the case after a good talk, people came up afterward and tried to catch the speaker for some additional questions. When his turn finally came, the distressed listener started asking questions that made it clear that for him, this was personal. In the end he explained that he was a successful anesthesiologist. In those days, that was a high-risk profession for developing opioid addiction because of easy access to morphine and less strict routines for controlling its use in hospitals than we have today.[2] After several years of morphine addiction, he had successfully kicked the habit, which is an impressive achievement. He had then worked for several years without relapsing. But Chuck's vivid description of the experimentally induced withdrawal had been enough of a cue for him to precipitate a powerful urge for morphine.

Patients and clinicians alike have long known that individuals with addictive disorders report craving and relapse when exposed to stimuli associated with their drug use, be that the street corner, the bar, or the drinking buddies. Understanding how these stimuli start playing an important role for triggering craving and relapse is probably one of the most important questions facing addiction research. Our ability to develop science-based therapies in part relies on our ability to understand mechanisms of cue-induced relapse and find ways of preventing this phenomenon from occurring. Abraham Wikler of the University of Kentucky is often credited with introducing the concept of conditioned drug cues as an important relapse factor, for instance, in a much cited paper from 1973.[3]. This initial proposition was based on clinical experience—some might say anecdotes—and theorizing. The *Science* paper by O'Brien and colleagues was the first scientific demonstration that the phenomenon postulated by Wikler actually happens in people. It was followed by work in the alcohol field carried out by Peter Monti at Brown University, who established that letting an alcohol-dependent patient handle and smell—but not consume—his or her preferred alcoholic beverage gave rise in a vast majority of patients to intense alcohol craving. Yet even after these demonstrations, it took a while before the importance of these findings was fully appreciated.

Unsurprisingly, the extinction–reinstatement model introduced in the previous chapter has also provided solid support for a critical role of drug-associated cues for relapse. Rats or other animals that have learned to self-administer drug in the presence of previously neutral stimuli and then undergone extinction will quickly resume lever pressing when they are reexposed to the drug-associated cues, much the same way as they do following a priming dose of the drug. This phenomenon is reliably reproduced for all major classes of addictive drugs, including alcohol. To date, many laboratories, including my own, rely on this model for our attempts to understand relapse induced by drug memories and the brain machinery that produces it. The model is also widely used in efforts to develop medications that could help prevent relapse triggered by drug or alcohol cues. In these experiments, we use cues that are very similar to those used in the original human experiments, such as a tone or an odor. The use of this animal model has allowed studies of brain circuitry that contributes to cue-induced relapse. A caveat is that most of the mapping studies have examined relapse to cocaine seeking. We do not know at this stage how similar the circuitry is for different drugs. Nevertheless, a part of the amygdala,[4] a structure in the temporal lobe that is critical for emotional aspects of learning, has through this work reliably been identified as a brain center that is critical for relapse triggered by drug-associated cues.

But we can't ask experimental animals whether they really crave drug when they run back to a lever and resume pressing it. At the same time, in attempting to identify the brain networks that produce subjective states such as craving in humans, research encounters two major obstacles. One is practical, the other conceptual. On a practical level, subjective states may be possible to assess in human subjects with addictive disorders through the use of carefully designed self-report measures, but not until recently did these studies allow an analysis of what brain circuitry generates the subjective states. Perhaps more important, many hard-nosed neuroscientists are inherently skeptical whether people can reliably report what is going on in their brains, such as craving, or causing their behavior, such as relapse. This is not to question the honesty of people who provide the self-reports; it is merely to consider the limits of our ability to look into our own brains.[5] Introspection may have fed an entire business of psychoanalysis but has simply not stood up to the test of science to provide us with an understanding of how the brain works to produce the mind. In the end, this is perhaps not entirely shocking. After all, you would not rely on introspection to find out if you have a brain tumor either, would you?

Advances in human functional brain imaging have to some extent helped break through these barriers. Using one of these imaging techniques, positron emission tomography, a groundbreaking paper in 1996 opened up a line of research that has since produced a convergence of human and animal studies.[6] That paper and many others that followed examined the relationship between cravings reported in response to drug cues and patterns of brain activity. In that study experienced cocaine users were shown videos of drug cues, such as white powder, a mirror, a razorblade, and a rolled-up dollar bill. Their responses were compared with those of research volunteers who had never used cocaine. As expected, showing the drug paraphernalia resulted in reports of powerful craving in the cocaine users but not in the participants who did not have experience with cocaine. The cocaine-user group also responded to the cocaine-related cues with increased brain activity, measured as consumption of sugar by nerve cells, which was visible in the PET images. Among the brain regions activated were parts of the frontal lobe and the amygdala,[7] which I have already mentioned is critical for emotional aspects of learning and memory. The greater the reports of craving, the greater the activity in these brain areas, the researchers found. In contrast, the volunteers who had never used cocaine and did not report cocaine cue-induced craving showed no signs of cue-induced brain activity in this area. Many similar studies have since followed, with increasingly sophisticated methodologies. Studies using both PET and fMRI have looked at the effects of drug-associated cues such as pictures of glasses or bottles with alcoholic beverages. Depending on the drug, experimental conditions, and study design, somewhat different patterns of network activations have been seen, but overall it seems clear that the subjective state of craving is associated with distinct changes in brain activity patterns. The intensity of these changes frequently correlates with the degree of craving.

The patterns that have emerged from the fMRI studies are slightly different from those initially suggested by the PET studies. This may be related to several things. As mentioned, the early PET studies employed sugar utilization to measure how nerve cell activity changed in response to the stimuli. Also, because of the nature of the method, the PET studies sum up data over a period of time that lasts many minutes. In contrast, fMRI studies rely for activity measures on how much of the oxygen nerve cells extract from blood and presumably use up. Because of that, these studies are able to measure second-to-second variation. One interesting study that used fMRI found that alcohol-associated cues, compared with cues that were neutral, resulted in activation of the nucleus accumbens, which is a key node of brain reward circuitry, as well as areas in the frontal lobes of the brain.[8] An important finding was that the magnitude of activation in these regions correlated with the subjective alcohol craving reported by alcohol-dependent patients. In contrast, no such correlation was found in social drinkers. This shows that the relationship between stimuli that elicit memories of alcohol use takes on a different role as alcoholism develops.

Other studies have shown that presentation of alcohol-associated pictures to alcoholics results in an enhanced activation of what is called the ventral visual stream. This is one of the two main brain networks that process visual information and is thought to deal with recognizing objects and representing their form. It has strong connections to the medial temporal lobe, which stores long-term memories, the limbic system, which controls emotions, and the dorsal visual stream, the other main vision network, which deals with object locations and motion. The increased activation of the ventral visual stream by alcohol-associated stimuli in alcoholics probably reflects that these visual cues have taken on an increased salience compared with other stimuli a person might attend to. And one classic regulator of assigning salience to things we see is our old friend the amygdala, which in part does so based on prior experience of those stimuli.

Overall the imaging studies have provided support for an involvement of a network of brain structures that include the amygdala, the insula, the nucleus accumbens, and parts of the frontal lobes in cue-induced cravings. That is in good agreement with available animal studies.[9] These insights are not only of academic interest. They are also potentially very useful in developing new addiction medications. If a medication can prevent the brain networks described here to become activated after exposure to drug cues, then chances are it will also be able to prevent cue-induced relapse. This approach to early drug development has the attraction that we can go by an objective measure rather than relying on subjective self-reports of patients.

And seeing is believing, isn't it? Not necessarily. The fact that a brain area lights up in conjunction with a particular behavior or experience does not necessarily mean that this brain area *causes* that behavior or experience. I cannot repeat enough times: correlation does not equal causation. This is the main weakness that plagues the exploding field of functional brain imaging, and the field of addiction research is no exception. But when brain imaging results converge with the results of animal studies in which we can isolate the causal role of a manipulation, then we can most likely gain important insights about mechanisms that cause rather than just correlate with addictive behaviors. That does seem to be the case with many of the studies on cue-induced craving and the brain networks that produce it.

In the future it may actually become possible to silence brain structures involved in representing drug memories and translating them into cravings and drug seeking. One approach that is of theoretical importance but is not likely to ever become a staple of clinical addiction medicine is deep brain stimulation (DBS). Rapidly adopted for the treatment of symptoms produced by Parkinson's disease, and more recently for obsessive-compulsive disorder and severe depression, this approach has been reported by a German group to dramatically reduce relapse when targeting one of the structures activated by drug-associated cues, the nucleus accumbens. This was observed in a small number of cases and could clearly be the result of a powerful placebo effect. But controlled studies are now under way and will allow data to be collected that can establish whether DBS actually causes an improvement in addictive disorders. A second approach that is being tried is much less invasive but also much blunter. Neurologists working on movement disorders have for some time known that sending a strong magnetic field into the brain, by placing a coil on the outside of the skull, can temporarily silence or stimulate underlying brain tissue. This method, called transcranial magnetic stimulation (TMS), can as effectively as innocently paralyze the thumb for a few minutes, demonstrating which part of the cerebral cortex produces thumb movements. The limitation until recently has been that the magnetic fields used have not been able to reach deeply enough into the brain to affect structures that are important for drug memories. Recent technological developments have, however, led to the construction of coils that can do just that. Studies on addictive disorders are currently ongoing using this approach, both to understand what brain structures do what and to prevent relapse.

Based on the developing understanding of how drug cues cause relapse, attempts have also been made to develop behavioral treatments. The principle is quite appealing. If the response to the drug cues could be extinguished in the lab, then perhaps the risk of craving and relapse upon encountering these cues in the real world could be decreased? It hasn't quite worked out that way. Yes, based on this expectation, Peter Monti and his colleagues developed "cue exposure therapy" (CET) for the treatment of alcoholism. Although the number of studies is still small, evidence from these controlled and well-designed trials does in fact support the notion that CET can reduce the frequency and severity of relapse.[10] I will revisit this approach in the chapter that discusses behavioral treatments for alcohol addiction. At this point, however, we should note two things. First, CET involves a considerably more sophisticated approach to relapse prevention than simply extinguishing cue-reactivity. Rather than relying on extinction alone, it involves teaching patients the coping skills needed to manage cravings that arise in response to alcohol cues without relapsing. Second, despite this thoughtful and rational approach, the effect size is modest.

One might wonder what is going on here. Presumably part of the answer is that cue-induced cravings are after all only one class of relapse triggers. Relapse in response to stress, which I will discuss next, is another major category and will not necessarily be affected by treatments that target cue-induced craving. Furthermore, some degree of drug sampling may occur in a mostly random fashion, or perhaps out of habit. This will effectively result in the delivery of priming drug doses, which we have already seen are powerful triggers for craving and relapse themselves.

But according to a hypothesis put forward by Yavin Shaham of NIDA, another important part of the answer may be related to the nature of the drug cues used in these procedures. There are different kinds of cues in the world around us. Some are discrete. In the artificial environment of the lab, the 700 Hz sound from the tone generator, played for a few seconds, is one of them. In the real world, the honking of a horn from a car might fall in the same category. Once one has learned to associate it with the image of a rapidly approaching car, a brief presentation will certainly be enough to make one step back to the curb. This kind of cue is simple in terms of what sensory modality it is picked up by, and it has a distinct onset and an equally distinct offset. But most cues that become associated with drug use in the real world, or for that matter with many other important processes, are far more complex. They provide an entire context in which the actions of the individual occur and with which they become associated—one that is woven from different strands of visual, auditory, tactile, and olfactory fabric. Accordingly, these cues are referred to as contextual.

The brain circuitry involved in relapse triggered by these two types of cues seems to be overlapping, but there are also important differences. As one might expect, the more complex contextual cues rely on a more widespread network of brain structures. In a parallel to what has been found in studies of learned fear, relapse triggered by discrete cues is for the most part related to the function of the amygdala and the nucleus accumbens. In contrast, relapse triggered by the more complex contextual cues in addition relies on another structure classically important for contextual learning and memory: the hippocampus.

It may well be that the more widespread brain networks that drive context-induced relapse inherently make this phenomenon harder to extinguish. But that aside, effectively extinguishing the right contextual cues in the laboratory is going to be difficult simply because the context is very different. The patient is in a hospital, not on the street. Around the patient are people whose looks, sounds, and smells are entirely different from those of people at a bar. I could go on and on, but you get the picture. It is clear that simulating and then extinguishing every possible context that may have become associated with using drugs or alcohol is a much more challenging task than simply extinguishing the response to a cue such as the look or smell of the alcoholic beverage itself. For all we know, the former task may pose a challenge that may simply turn out to be insurmountable. Whether that is going to be the case will obviously be a matter of research, not of opinion.

A fascinating recent development offers some hope that another psychological approach may circumvent the challenges outlined above. Rather than attempting to induce new learning that would extinguish drug responses to drug cues in every conceivable situation, this approach attempts to erase them. This research is based on major discoveries in the field of fear learning, which for many years has provided some of the best models to study how memories are made and unmade. In an extreme oversimplification, memories are first acquired, in an unstable form, into working memory that uses parts of the frontal lobes. They are then consolidated with the help of parts of the amygdala and the hippocampus. Once consolidation has occurred, they are available to be retrieved in response to the right cue or context. But about a decade ago, Karim Nader, now at McGill University, and his mentor at the time, Joseph LeDoux at New York University,[11] provided provocative data in support of an additional process, called reconsolidation. The idea is that when a memory trace is retrieved, it transiently becomes unstable, just as it was originally, and will now require reconsolidation to be stored once more. Manipulations during a critical time window following retrieval, while the memory trace is still unstable, will prevent its reconsolidation, essentially making the memory go away.[12] Recently this procedure was applied to relapse behavior in rats and drug craving in heroin addicts, in both cases triggered by drug-associated cues. Both in rats and in people, the appropriate manipulation during the time window of reconsolidation seemed to eliminate the behavioral responses to the respective cues, much the way it has been able to erase learned fear responses.[13] If replicated, this approach clearly holds the promise to add an important tool to the treatment toolkit and help prevent relapse triggered by drug memories.

Those psychologically inclined may find it appealing to work on designing therapies that will extinguish responses to multiple, varying contexts, hoping that the extinction process will somehow generalize, or erase drug memories altogether. These are reasonable, promising approaches to addressing the challenge of cue-induced relapse. I certainly hope for them to be successful. For the more neuropharmacologically inclined scientists, it might instead be appealing to think that there is a final common pathway through which different types of cues promote relapse. If that final common pathway uses specific transmitters and receptors, then blocking the function of these might hold the same kind of promise. What the outcome will be is a purely empirical question. I don't care much who "wins," as long as we get something that works. As will we will see in a coming chapter, there is evidence that a pharmacological approach might hold some promise as well.

12

A STRAINED MIND

I T IS TWELVE noon on a scorching weekday in the summer. You are stationed at the Miramar Naval Air Base outside San Diego. It is your day off, and you and your comrades are driving to the beach. Pete is driving, and you are in the passenger seat. Phil, Matt, Bob, and Chris are in the back. You narrow your eyes to block out the blazing sun. Suddenly you smell smoke. Your heart quickens. You drive a little farther and see an accident about 150 yards away. You tense the muscles in your face and forehead. You think, "My God, has a plane gone down?" You move in closer and see a sedan that has collided with a white van. The muscles in your back and shoulders become tense. You notice that the front end of the car is completely smashed in. The van has flipped over on the passenger's side. By now, your heart is racing. You pile out of the vehicle and break up into teams. You see a balding male in his thirties in the front seat of the sedan. The crown of his head is stuck in the windshield and the column of the steering wheel has impaled his neck. You feel nauseous. He is groaning and his eyelids are flickering. You think, "This is hopeless." You tense the muscles in your back, arms, and legs. You hear muffled cries. Your eyes glance over at the van. Black smoke is swirling up from it. You clench your jaw. You think, "We have to get those people out before it blows." Your breathing becomes faster. You run over to the van and look inside. You see an adult male, a female, an infant, and three toddlers trapped inside. You feel hot all over. You see the mother slumped over and stretching her arms toward the infant on the floor. She is hysterical and screaming in Spanish. Your heart is pounding. Phil appears with a fire extinguisher and hoses down the van. One of your comrades uses a crowbar to break the windows and pry open the doors. Another hoists the father out of the van. You hold onto his upper torso. You can see that his back is contorted. You grit your teeth. The smell of gasoline is overpowering. You are drenched in sweat. You place the father's body on the ground away from the van. The mother is almost completely covered in a dark green rebozo, but you can see bone protruding through the bloody flesh of her left wrist, and her right arm is mangled. You tense the muscles all over your body. The toddlers are extracted but are dazed and pale. Your heart is racing. Pete, Phil, and Matt lift the mother out and lay her on the ground next to her husband. Your mouth feels parched. Pete slides half his body back into the van and hands you the infant, who looks like a tiny doll. It feels fragile and almost weightless in your hands. Bright red blood is all over its little, round face and running out of its mouth. Your whole body is tense. You hear it making small, quick, raspy breaths. You think, "It is still alive!" Suddenly the breaths cease and the baby goes limp. A cold chill cascades down your spine. You place your head to its mouth and feel for a pulse on the neck with your fingers. There is no pulse! Your hands tremble. You perform CPR but there is no response. You feel helpless. You think, "No, no, this can't be happening. This baby is innocent. It can't be dead!" There is a lump in your throat. There is nothing you can do to change this. You want to scream and strike someone. There is a deep, intense pain sensation inside.[1]

The account above is based on an interview that was carried out with one of our research patients, who suffered from the all too common combination of posttraumatic stress disorder (PTSD) and alcoholism, shortly after he was admitted to the unit. Following the interview, a standardized procedure was used to develop the script, which one of our research nurses read and recorded. The recording takes about five minutes. It was played back to the patient a couple of weeks later. It is easy to imagine the intense emotional distress it made the patient feel. It is less obvious that listening to this script would also give rise to an intense craving for alcohol. Yet that is one of the most striking consequences when these stress scripts are presented to our alcohol-addicted patients. The cravings are not only intense, they also continue for a surprisingly long time. Although the presentation only lasts five minutes, it takes more than an hour and a half before the cravings subside.

PTSD is of course the extreme of stress. But patients and clinicians alike have long held that stress exposure is a major factor behind craving and relapse to alcohol use. Alan Marlatt, the father of psychological relapse prevention treatment, listed stressors among relapse triggers about which patients with alcoholism need to be educated. One of the main tenets of this treatment approach was that patients need to develop coping strategies to eliminate stressors from their lives if possible, or otherwise develop and practice strategies to cope with them without relapsing to alcohol use. Yet for a long time there has also been a considerable ambivalence both within the research community and outside it toward acknowledging the critical role of stress as a relapse factor. This is in part understandable. After all, there is almost invariably some unpleasant experience that a relapse could be blamed on after it has occurred. It is hard to know what causes what in the complicated web of real life. And the last thing we want is to promote a perception among patients that they are helpless victims of external circumstances.

By now, however, two parallel developments have firmly established the role of stress as a critically important relapse factor in addictive disorders. One of these developments is an accumulation of data obtained by studying responses to stressful provocations in the laboratory, perhaps most successfully through the approach I just illustrated. Guided imagery, as this approach is called, is a powerful method to induce vivid recollections of highly stressful personal experiences and the emotional states with which they were associated. This is not just a dry retelling of a stressful event. One key to the power of this methodology is that it goes beyond the external events that made up the experience. It also takes great care to obtain from the subject a detailed account of the bodily responses that the external events produced. Note, for instance, in the script describing the nightmare of the car accident the descriptions of the subject's heart pounding, his muscles becoming tense, and his body becoming hot.

This methodology, first developed in other areas of psychology, was brought to addiction research by Raijta Sinha of Yale University, a clinical psychologist and one of the most creative and successful contemporary scientists studying the role of stress for craving and relapse. In a series of papers published over the past decade, Rajita has shown that exposure to stress scripts like these reliably and potently induces cravings in patients with addictive disorders. Her Yale team has by now shown this with patients addicted to different classes of drugs, including cocaine and alcohol. Other stressors have also been used in this kind of research. Using these approaches, other scientists have identified an important difference between patients with addictive disorders and social drinkers who are addicted to alcohol. Both groups respond with emotional distress to the stress challenge, but is only in people with alcoholism is this accompanied by alcohol craving. Once more we see evidence that the brain changes in the course of developing alcohol addiction, creating a connection between stress and the motivation to seek and consume alcohol.

The fact that alcohol-addicted patients crave in response to stress exposure is interesting but does not on its own establish a connection between those cravings and relapse risk. What the Yale group has demonstrated, in a major advance for the field, is that the intensity of the craving response to stress exposure really predicts the risk for relapse over a subsequent period of time, after the patient has been discharged from the hospital. They have shown that this holds true for cocaine addiction as well.[2] This work and similar results obtained by others provide strong support for a relationship between stress-induced craving and relapse. Those findings are also a big help for research that is aimed at improving treatment of addictive disorders. Full-scale treatment trials require hundreds of patients and long follow-up times. They are therefore very expensive, and only a small number of particularly promising medications can be tested using this approach.[3] But if craving responses to stress in the laboratory tell us something about relapse risk, then laboratory experiments offer a tool to sift through potential medications and select those for which the investment of a full-scale treatment study may be justified. Several medications are currently being evaluated using this approach.

In an appealing convergence of clinical and basic research, scientists have also found that stress triggers resumption of drug and alcohol seeking in animal experiments. To recap, this research often uses the model in which animals are trained to lever press for a drug but then have this behavior extinguished by changing the rules so that pressing the lever no longer results in drug delivery. After extinction, stress will make the animal run back to the lever that previously delivered the drug and resume lever pressing. Although stimuli that reinstate drug seeking in this way are the same for different drugs, such as alcohol, cocaine, and heroin, there are also interesting differences. For instance, priming with a small drug dose, discussed in a prior chapter, is a potent trigger for resumption of cocaine seeking. In contrast, priming is only modestly effective when it comes to alcohol. Stress, however, is uniformly potent in triggering relapse to drug seeking, irrespective of drug category.

By studying the brain circuits that produce stress-induced relapse in animals, scientists hope to discover new ways through which medications can help prevent relapse in patients with addictive disorders. Based on this type of research, several promising mechanisms are undergoing clinical evaluation. Perhaps the most important among these are blockers of a receptor for the main brain mediator of stress responses, corticotropin releasing factor (CRF).[4]

The existence of CRF was predicted many years prior to its actual discovery. This was based on a principle for which Roger Guillemin and Andrew Schally came to share the Nobel Prize in Medicine or Physiology already in 1977. Until the late 1950s the pituitary gland, a small structure that looks a bit like an upside-down mushroom and is located just under the base of the skull, was considered the "master gland" of the body. The name seemed justified because the pituitary secretes hormones that travel through the bloodstream and control hormone production by glands that are the business end of the respective hormonal axis—the thyroid, the sex glands, and the adrenals. But in the late 1950s scientists began to realize that the brain itself must be the real "master gland." It became clear that a part of the brain located at its base, the hypothalamus, must be sending signals to the pituitary and using these signals to control hormone production. For many years these signals remained purely hypothetical and were therefore referred to as hypothalamic factors. Guillemin and Schally initially collaborated on trying to find these mythical substances but ultimately became engaged in a fierce competition. They ended up independently isolating the first hypothalamic releasing factor at about the same time. With this discovery, the control of the thyroid gland became understood, and the mythical "thyrotropin releasing factor" become a real thing, whose molecular structure you could draw, and which you could make in the lab. With that, it also became elevated to the status of a real hormone, reflected in the name thyrotropin releasing hormone (TRH).

But when Guillemin and Schally went to Stockholm to receive their Nobel for the discovery of TRH, an important hypothalamic releasing factor was still missing and was the subject of a furiously competitive search. When the organism is faced with a major challenge, it must mobilize all its resources to cope. To accomplish this, the pituitary sends adrenocorticotropic hormone (ACTH) to the adrenals. In response, the adrenals secrete cortisol, the main stress hormone of the body. Cortisol then does most of the things classically associated with the stress response. For instance, it instructs the liver and muscles to open up their stores of sugar and send glucose out as fuel into the bloodstream. At the same time, it turns off long-term processes, such as the buildup of proteins, which clearly can wait until the acute threat has been handled.[5] There is, after all, little point to building up your muscles for tomorrow if you don't survive the attack of the saber-toothed tiger today.

But if the brain is the master gland, then the hypothalamus must be releasing a factor that controls ACTH secretion from the pituitary in response to stress. Together with ACTH and cortisol, this hypothetical signal would form the cascade that became known as the hypothalamic-pituitary-adrenal (HPA) axis, a critically important system for coping with stress.[6] The discovery of CRF as the master controller of the HPA axis is the subject of its own scientific legend. An exceptionally talented young scientist, Wylie Vale, trained as a postdoctoral fellow with Guillemin at the Salk Institute in La Jolla. When he started his own lab at the Salk, several other brilliant scientists, as well as one of the most skilled technicians from his old mentor's lab, followed him. The legend has it that Vale and his stellar team raced his Nobel-winning former mentor for the discovery of the mythical CRF molecule. He got there first and was able to publish its isolation in the journal *Science* in 1981.[7] It turned out to be a small protein, or a "peptide," made from forty-one amino acids that are the building blocks of proteins.

This finding, one of the classics of physiology, was greeted with great excitement by the entire field of endocrinology, the study of hormones, their regulation, and their effects on the body. It sparked a line of research that continues to be a major success story to the present day. But just as important was the discovery that followed: that CRF is present not only in the hypothalamus but also in many other brain centers. These seemed to have little to do with hormonal responses. George Koob, one of the towering figures of modern addiction research whom we have already met in this book, became an early collaborator of Vale's. He showed that CRF in these "extrahypothalamic" brain regions controls the behavioral and emotional components of the stress response, which act in concert with, but separately from, the effects on metabolism and other body functions. CRF in the HPA axis will make sure that resources in the body are redirected to make fuel available to cope with the threat. CRF in extrahypothalamic brain areas will initiate the various behaviors that make up the coping response and will use that fuel. Research over the past three decades has shown that blocking actions of CRF prevents a wide range of these behavioral stress responses.

Increasing recognition that stress plays an important role in relapse to drug seeking, combined with an understanding that CRF plays a major role for behavioral stress responses, prompted the question whether CRF may also play a role in promoting relapse. In the late 1990s the laboratory of Yavin Shaham, then still in Toronto, could show just that. CRF receptor blockers prevented stress-induced relapse to heroin seeking. Shortly thereafter Anh Lê, working in collaboration with Yavin, found that CRF_1 receptor blockers also potently prevent relapse to alcohol seeking. Others showed that CRF_1 blockers may have potential to complement treatment with the clinically approved alcoholism medication naltrexone. This was because in experimental animals, CRF_1 blockade prevented stress-induced relapse but not relapse triggered by alcohol cues. The effects of naltrexone were just the opposite: it blocked relapse in response to alcohol cues but not in response to stress. The combination of naltrexone and a CRF_1 blocker prevented relapse whether triggered by a drug cue or by stress. Because relapse in the real world is triggered by both stressors and drug cues, the two treatments should have potential to be complementary and additive in clinical treatment as well. In subsequent studies several laboratories, including ours, have shown that different blockers of CRF_1 receptors all have the ability to prevent stress-induced relapse. Clinical studies are now ongoing to establish whether this translates into an ability to prevent stress-induced cravings in patients with alcohol addiction.

Because of the fundamental role the HPA axis response and cortisol play for physiology and coping with stress, it is tempting to jump to the conclusion that the ability of CRF blockers to prevent stress-induced relapse is related to their ability to prevent HPA axis activation and resulting cortisol production. Actually, that is *not* how it works. In laboratory experiments the adrenals can be removed and their production of corticosterone, the rat equivalent of cortisol, replaced by a pellet that will provide the animal with a constant level of this hormone. After this manipulation, there is no longer an HPA axis activation in response to stress. The cortisol levels are flat no matter what happens. Yet this manipulation will not influence stress-induced relapse. At the same time, CRF_1 blockers will still be effective to prevent stress-induced relapse under these conditions. Clearly CRF blockers must produce their effect through actions outside the HPA axis, in "extrahypothalamic" brain areas. It turns out that, to a large extent, the anti-relapse effects of CRF blockers happen in the amygdala. This makes perfect sense since parts of the amygdala are potently activated by the same types of stressors that also reliably induce relapse to drug seeking.

CRF_1 blockers are promising as a future alcoholism treatment but have taken many years to reach evaluation in patients. First, it was difficult for the medicinal chemists to develop blockers with the right properties, such as uptake from the stomach and into the brain. Once that was finally achieved, interest from the drug industry was primarily directed toward treatment of anxiety and depression, where results have been disappointing for reasons that are still unclear. Addiction treatment is unfortunately at the bottom of the totem pole for the industry, so it was only after failures in depression and anxiety that CRF_1 blockers became available for evaluation in addictive disorders. Those studies are ongoing. Answers will be in within the next couple of years. Given all the years of research behind these trials, it is both an exciting and a scary time to be in this field.

I am reasonably hopeful that CRF_1 blockers may become important additions to the treatment toolkit, but drug development really is a gamble. Medications with the best possible basic science support still run a high risk of failing. This can sometimes be because of differences between our basic science models and the clinical condition. But failures are also common for reasons that have nothing to do with science and may appear trivial, such as unacceptable side effects in some completely unrelated organ. So it is important that we don't bet all our chips on any single mechanism and instead maintain a pipeline of medication candidates. Several other anti-stress mechanisms hold promise to prevent stress-induced relapse and are being pursued by different laboratories. As we will see in a bit, different medications may turn out to be helpful for different patients. There will never be a magic bullet. The hope is that there will be incremental advances and personalized treatments.

The way basic and clinical research has converged to support the notion that stress is critically important for relapse to alcohol seeking is indeed encouraging. As we have seen, this convergence promises to help scientists develop new medications for alcoholism and other addictions. But there are clearly important limitations to the similarities between laboratory rodents and people. For instance, stressors that most effectively trigger relapse to drug seeking are very different for different species. In the rat experiments scientists are most successful using simple physical stressors. Mild electric shocks, administered through the grid of the cage floor for about ten minutes, work best. This may seem artificial but may actually make sense from the perspective of a rat. After all, if you are a rat, most threats in the environment are of a physical nature, frequently represent immediate threats to survival, and are signaled by aversive sensations such as pain.

Over the course of evolution, the situation has become very different for social, group-living primates, with their elaborate social structures and long-lasting attachment bonds. Among these species, an individual's place in the social hierarchy, success or failure in establishing alliances with other members of the troop, and stability of the social order are the most important stressors. Survival depends to a large extent on successful social adjustment. We humans are of course one of these primate species, and the development toward an increasingly important role of social factors as stressors has clearly reached an entirely new level in human societies. The account of events at the beginning of the chapter certainly serves as a reminder that physical threats to survival by no means have been eliminated from our lives. But it is also clear that this type of experience represents an extreme, and one that becomes less and less frequent in affluent, well-organized societies. In many ways, success in shielding us from hunger, disease, and physical threat has come both thanks to but also at the expense of ever-increasing social complexity and demands on social adjustment.

And so in fact most stressors that lead to relapse in patients with addictive disorders are of a social nature. The classic triggers reported over and over again by countless patients are antagonistic encounters with a spouse, a friend, or a boss. These situations signal powerful social threats. They indicate the possibility of disruption to attachment bonds on which our family universe and its protection of offspring relies for its existence, through which our needs for social support outside the family are met, or through which we fit into a context that promises to ensure continued provision of resources for sustaining us and our offspring.

For many years, research on the web of an individual's social relationships and that on the function of the brain seemed to live in different worlds. It was hard to imagine how that gap could be bridged. A highly original line of research by Naomi Eisenberger, a psychologist and brain imager at University of California, Los Angeles, provides a template for how that kind of synthesis can be achieved. In a landmark paper Eisenberger and colleagues were able to model social rejection inside an fMRI camera.[8] They used a seemingly simple task called cyberball. In this task the subjects are asked to play a computer game that involves passing a ball around between players. They are told that they are playing with other participants over a computer network. In fact, however, there are no other participants. There is just the computer program. For the first few rounds, the ball is indeed passed around, but after a while the other "players" begin to omit the participant. One would think that this would be a rather innocent form of social exclusion, but participants become visibly upset. Being able to model some of the feelings triggered by rejection in the laboratory made it possible to study what brain networks produce them. The astounding observation was that during rejection, a brain network was activated that was already well familiar to scientists. Its activation had previously been described many times in subjects who experience physical pain. Hence the title of the paper: "Does Rejection Hurt?"

One of the main nodes in the pain network activated by the cyberball task is called the insula. This is a region of cerebral cortex that dates back to early stages of human evolution and is folded deep within the lateral groove between the temporal and frontal lobe. The insula has a unique role in apes and humans, in that it encodes unpleasant feelings that arise from the inside of the body, such as nausea. But as we know from expressions such as "gut feeling" or "gut-wrenching experience," many stressors give rise to similar unpleasant bodily states.

The relationship between social rejection as a stressor, on one hand, and craving and relapse, on the other, has not yet been directly established. But I have already noted that rejection activates the insula. At the same time, functional brain imaging studies have shown that the insula is activated when people report drug or alcohol cravings, and the intensity of this activation often correlates with how intensely the cravings are experienced. Again, correlation does not necessarily equal causation. But in studying another addiction, that to nicotine, an unusually elegant paper showed that brain damage affecting the insula effectively eliminated cigarette cravings and helped patients quit smoking.[9] Based on these various observations, it is tempting to speculate what might be going on: development of alcohol addiction leads to an exaggerated insula response to social stress and contributes to relapse by translating that response into a feeling of craving. Although evidence for this chain of events is not yet fully in place, a French group recently demonstrated that the insula response to rejection in the cyberball task is indeed greater in people with alcoholism.[10]

At this point it is worthwhile to lift our outlook beyond the closely controlled laboratory experiments and consider more broadly what addiction does in the social domain. Obviously the more drug seeking takes over a patient's life, the less the ability of the individual to pursue goals that are shared with others, to function in a social context, and to engage in all the things necessary for successful membership in a modern society. This leads to progressive social exclusion and marginalization, a process that ultimately takes on a life of its own for most patients with more severe forms of addictions, in the form of family disruption, joblessness, and lack of other sources of social support. But marginalization is in turn, as we have seen, a potent social stressor. So of course it feeds increased motivation for drug seeking and relapse. This vicious circle is hard to break. It will obviously require a lot more than medications to do so. But medications that can reduce cravings triggered by social stress will be an important component in successful rehabilitation.

13

FATHERS AND SONS

THE CALLER, A father of two boys, was a leading Swedish industrialist. People spoke of him as a good man, but even so, I found these referrals somewhat awkward. Most of our patients were disadvantaged; many were homeless. All had neglected medical needs. I had mixed feelings about treating or advising people who had vast resources available to them, and who expected us to give them special attention. We just didn't do VIP treatment. When the caller asked if I could please see him and his sons in my private practice, I explained I didn't have one. He insisted he could not be seen at the clinic with his sons. It was a simple statement of fact: they would not come with him. Could I please see them somewhere else? I apologized and said the clinic was the one place where I saw patients. He insisted. This would actually not be about treatment at all, he promised; it was just that his family needed advice. He thought maybe his youngest son in particular would find it easier to receive that from a stranger than from his father. I quietly thought back to my own father and the stormy years until he became my best friend. I guess I could relate. And I did of course have an office in our home on the outskirts of Stockholm, where I tried to write scientific papers at night, after the kids had fallen asleep. It would have to do.

As I was greeting them, I was struck by what a curious trio they were. The father, a commanding man in his fifties, blond with a bit of gray here and there, was still strikingly fit. He dressed with simple, understated elegance, and it was easy to see what a forceful presence he could be. But at the time, he was measured, almost restrained. After he introduced himself and his sons, he sat down and let them do the talking. The older son, on the Swedish national track and field team, had the cliché looks of an elite athlete. In this case that basically meant a younger version of his dad, with more muscle but the same quiet, restrained energy. It was the younger son who drew the most attention. Thinner than the other two men, fidgety and visibly less confident, he clearly found the situation awkward and took every chance to monkey around just to relieve the tension. His older brother looked embarrassed, and the jokes really were juvenile. But it was also clear that this was a sweet guy who adored his big brother and had tremendous respect for his father.

In a way the story was quite simple. Both sons were exceptional track-and-field talents, recognized as such from their youngest years, and fulfilling the promise at every stage. Good genes, I remember thinking. Their father, it turned out, had been a promising college athlete, too, before engineering and business studies, and then running a rapidly expanding company, set him on a different path. Over the course of the conversation, I learned that he still beat both of his sons at tennis and still did the classic Swedish cross-country ski race, Vasaloppet, which runs over a distance of 56 miles every winter. The older son was about to face the decision his father had once had to make—whether to pursue a career as an athlete and try to become competitive at an international level or to keep the good memories and focus on getting his engineering degree. He seemed to slowly be getting ready for the latter alternative but wasn't there quite yet. The younger son was at a very different point. He was only now approaching the junction when he would reveal his true potential, as the junior team was occasionally invited to join the national team for training camps, and the coaches scouted for talent. Except every time that happened, things went terribly wrong. After the hard workouts, they partied. And every time they partied, this pleasant, polite young man drank everyone else under the table and did crazy things. On one occasion he would get into a fight over something silly; on another, he would walk out on a bridge, get up on the handrail, and do a balancing act 30 feet up in the air that only luck prevented from ending with a fatal outcome.

As I started to piece together the family history, the picture was clear. It had not been talked about much in the family, but the grandfather, an army officer, must have been an alcoholic. The father had decided to stay away from alcohol at a young age, while himself in the military service. Prior to that decision, there had been some episodes that involved crazy use of firearms but fortunately didn't end with a tragedy. One day the young man who would become the father of the two boys in front of me decided never again to touch alcohol, and he kept that promise ever since. He had not talked with his sons about this experience until the older one tried alcohol around the age of eighteen and came to him, troubled by his own reaction. The two were very close. After a long conversation with his father, the older boy started a determined effort to practice skills that helped him handle drinking, much the way he would have practiced a new high-jump technique. He would still take the occasional glass but learned to stop at that. And for the most part, he just told people that alcohol would spoil some special training regimen he was following. That was hard to argue with. But his younger brother did not seem willing or able to master those kinds of tools. He just wanted to be one of the boys, like his big brother. And now he was about to be kicked off the team because of bad behavior.

I explained what we knew about how and why alcoholism risk runs in families. Thankfully the older two men had the good sense to keep quiet, sometimes nodding to affirm some of the things I said, sometimes just asking a clarifying question. I basically summarized what they had told me and put it in a broader context. The younger son stopped fidgeting and listened. After a while he became visibly upset and actually quite hostile. I shrugged it off. "Look, it's not your fault and it's not mine," I said. "People are born certain ways and can neither take credit nor be blamed for it. You are blond and my hair is dark. I'll never run 200 meters under 22 seconds, and you will always have a hard time controlling your alcohol reactions. It is not a big deal. But whether you like it or not, you are the one who will have to live with it." His anger dissipated and turned into a sadness that for a while filled the room. We were quiet and let it sink in. As he started asking questions, it was a very different, subdued, more mature person talking. At some point I could also see curiosity take over. "How does it work?" he asked. I summarized some of the key studies. I also told him all the things we still did not know.

The young man had some unusual resources available to him. Like his father and his older brother, he was very smart. He also had their experience to relate to. He thought things were unfair, but he also realized that Mother Nature did not care much about his opinion in the matter. He got it, he said. But what if he still wasn't ready to completely give up drinking? he asked. Would I still have some useful advice to offer him?

Everybody in the addiction field knows what to say in response at this point: "Young man, you have not yet fully accepted that you are powerless under your addiction and poor you until you do." Except this guy was not even an alcoholic, at least not yet. And this was around the time we were beginning to figure out some things that challenged conventional wisdom. We already knew, for instance, from analyses that pooled results from many different controlled clinical studies, that a strong family history of alcoholism was a sign people had a better than average chance of responding well to naltrexone. Of course, the approved use of naltrexone was to take the medication every day. For someone who drank only a few times a year, that just didn't seem reasonable.

I don't know what got into me. I said, "You really should follow your father's example. See how well he has done with his decision. But until you are ready to do that, here is something else we can try, almost as an experiment. I'll write you a naltrexone prescription. When you absolutely want to go to a party where there is a chance you will use alcohol, take the medication a couple of hours ahead of time. Then come see me three months from now, at the clinic, and tell me how you are doing. And call us if you get in any kind of trouble." He nodded quietly. I followed him for about two years. He relapsed to heavy drinking once. After more than a year of controlled and seemingly harmless alcohol use, he decided he was probably cured and tried to skip the medication. Next time, he drank himself to a blackout, fought with his best friend without later being able to recall over what, and ended up in a police cell. By the time he came back for an appointment to tell me about it all, he had already returned to the medication, and things were back on track.

Then, after about two more years of follow-up, he said he no longer needed to come back. I worried about him, but as he was leaving my office, he gave me a funny smile and reassured me. Half a year later he sent me a letter. In it he thanked me and explained why he no longer needed my help. He was close to twenty-one now. He had come to realize that when he drank without being on naltrexone, he was walking a tightrope over the abyss and would sooner or later fall. When he drank on naltrexone, it was pretty much pointless, with none of the bright light flooding his mind, and the most prominent result instead being headaches. As he was mulling over his options, he had encountered the old Mark Twain quote: "When I was a boy of fourteen, my father was so ignorant I could hardly stand to have the old man around. But when I got to be twenty-one, I was astonished at how much the old man had learned in seven years." He talked to his father. After a series of conversations, he decided that for them, drinking was just not an option.

Alcoholism runs in families. Laura Bierut, a leading genetic epidemiologist of addiction at Washington University, St. Louis, likes to remind her audiences that this insight is in many ways unremarkable. Already the ancient Greeks seem to have attributed a significant part of alcoholism risk to genetics. Aristotle wrote that "drunken women bring forth children like themselves,"[1] while Plutarch stated that "one drunkard begets another." Some two thousand years later, similar observations were noted in Scandinavian church books, one of the best-preserved sources of multigenerational family history information recorded to this time. In the margins of those books, notes can frequently be found from long forgotten ministers describing how drunkenness had run in a family for generations. Interestingly, that insight never seems to have prevented those ministers from preaching that the drunkard could and should change his ways. Clearly, in their mind, acknowledging a genetic influence did not imply a view of genes as destiny.

The fact that alcoholism and other addictions run in families does not, on its own, prove that there is a substantial genetic component to the risk for developing these disorders. It could well be that the risk, for the most part at least, instead comes from growing up in a family affected by addictive disorders. Other shared environmental factors, outside the family, could contribute too. Addiction is after all strongly associated with growing up and living in poverty, being exposed to violence, or having a low level of education. Each or all of these factors could theoretically contribute to addiction risk. Whether most of the risk comes from genes, the shared environmental factors, or a combination of the two is therefore an empirical question. Simply stated, good-quality data about the world are needed to decide it. It cannot be settled on the basis of one view being more appealing than the other. Nor is it helpful to consider which view is more in line with an enlightened political agenda. Yet that is exactly how smart, well-educated, and well-meaning people for a long time argued about these matters.

In short, for decades the argument of progressive intellectuals and their followers was that acknowledging a role of heritable, biological factors for complex behaviors such as drug seeking and excessive drug use leads to "a reductionist, biological determinist explanation of human existence. Its adherents claim, first, that the details of present and past social arrangements are the inevitable manifestations of the specific action of genes."[2]

Amazingly, world-class scientists such as the Harvard evolutionary biologist Richard Lewontin helped lend credence to this type of argument, and the quote above is in fact from a book Lewontin coauthored. For a long time those of us who dreamed of improved conditions for poor, disadvantaged, and addicted people were expected to subscribe to the notion that the human mind must start out as Locke's blank slate,[3] fully malleable by society's influence.[4] Only that would be compatible with progress. Anything else, and in particular considering an important role for inherited biological factors, rapidly qualified one for a label as a reactionary.

This was very peculiar, even as a hypothesis, for several reasons. First, humans have since the dawn of written history known that physical traits such as size have a strong genetic influence. For instance, we have long known and made use of the fact that domestic animals can be bred for those traits. A chihuahua will not grow into a mastiff no matter how much it is fed. But just like breeding large dogs and small dogs, we have also bred watchdogs that are territorial and aggressive, as well as child-loving black labs that will happily lick burglars all the way to the door when they leave with their loot. So to claim that there could not be a genetic influence on temperament or other complex behavioral traits would require that humans somehow be fundamentally different in their genetic transmission or their brain function from all other mammalian species. That is a claim for which there has never been a basis.

Second, the very reason physicians like myself want to know about genetic risk factors is that we think they may offer our patients means to intervene and change potentially devastating outcomes. Consider if your grandfather, your father, and your brother all got in trouble with alcohol, and if, on first trying alcohol, you experienced that you could drink more than anyone and enjoy it. Would you under those circumstances not want to consider the possibility that there is something about the response to alcohol running in your family that puts you at risk? But if you realized that to be the case, decided alcohol is just too dangerous for someone with your disposition, and stopped using it, you would radically change your fate, would you not? Or maybe, in the age of personalized medicine, you would instead decide to use a medication that prevented that enjoyable reaction to alcohol, allowing you to avoid the risk that way. Now, how is that for "biological determinism"?

There is in fact nothing deterministic about understanding the influence of genes for behavior. Knowledge is power. As every reader of Percy Jackson knows, *gnothi seauton* is the first advice the Oracle has to offer anyone on a quest to achieve something difficult and important.

Having said that, it is not a trivial task to parse out the contribution to addiction risk from genes, on one hand, and environmental factors, on the other. It is even harder to find the specific genes that contribute to the genetic risk. As we will see in the following, the past thirty years or so have seen some remarkable scientific advances in the former domain. Converging conclusions have been reached using quite different and complementary scientific methods. While each of those may have its weaknesses and potential sources of error, those sources are different for the different methods. The convergence therefore makes it highly probable that the conclusions are correct. I will in a moment explain in more detail what that statement means, and also, importantly, what it does not mean. The fundamental issue is, however, largely settled: addictive disorders are all moderately to highly heritable.

The other set of questions, prompted by that conclusion, has turned out to be much harder. What characteristics are being inherited that put people at risk for addiction? And what are the gene variants that contribute to the heritability of addiction that research has established? How many of those variants does it take for a significant level of risk—a few, a few hundred, a few thousand? We don't know, but it looks like it might be more than many of us thought just ten years ago. Progress in finding these risk variants has been frustrating, but there are advances in that area as well.

Umeå, home to Sweden's northernmost medical school, is located about 250 miles south of the polar circle, but you wouldn't know it from the weather. As far as the climate is concerned, this could just as well be the North Pole. The saying goes, if you survive the first winter, maybe you'll stay, but most people don't. By the time I met him some fifteen years ago, Michael Bohman had long retired as chair of child psychiatry in Umeå, had moved back to his native Stockholm, and was mostly pursuing his literary interests.

It was only when I actually met him that I realized Michael had started out as a psychoanalytically trained child psychiatrist. As a young physician, he told me, he had taken for granted the psychoanalytic teaching that early life experiences shape people's lives in major ways. He got involved in adoption studies because that line of research seemed to offer a promising way of finding out about the influence of early family environment and parsing it out from any genetic factors. In principle, if early family environment was influential the way psychoanalytic teachings had hypothesized, then various behaviors of children who were adopted early in life should be more influenced by their adoptive than their biological parents. Michael realized, as many genetic epidemiologists have since, that Sweden offers unique opportunities for this kind of research. Say what you will about the social democratic welfare state, but Sweden is sure good at keeping track of people, from birth to the grave. After all, how else would we know where to send all those welfare checks to everybody?

Michael collected the data for the Stockholm Adoption Study before landing his faculty position and moving north, but he continued to work on them after the move. The study, he wrote in a 1981 paper,

> was suitable for cross-fostering analysis because it involves a large population in which there has been no selection among the adoptees for particular types of parents or children. The population includes all persons born out of wedlock in Stockholm from 1930 through 1949 and placed for adoption. Most of the children were separated from their biological relatives in the first few months of life. The average age at final placement in the adoptive home was 8 months. Sweden is an ideal site for an adoption study. Extensive social and medical records about the adoptees and their parents have been obtained from several public sources by Bohman and his associates. Alcohol is readily available for consumption, but its abuse is under rather intense social sanction. A Temperance Board in each community is legally responsible to maintain sobriety. This board imposes fines for intemperance and supervises the treatment of alcoholics. Other records about diagnoses and treatment are kept by agencies of the National Health Insurance.
>
> In contrast, in the United States, records about biological parents obtained by adoption agencies are often incomplete and limited to the period prior to adoption, which usually occurs when the biological parents are quite young and not through the age of risk for psychiatric illness. The availability of objective and systematic lifetime data in Sweden avoids the potentially serious biases inherent in assessments based on self-report.[5]

It was clear that the data collected through the Stockholm Adoption Study were unique, but Bohman and his collaborator Sigvardsson, a psychologist, were initially struggling to make sense of them. The results simply did not seem to fit their hypothesis by any stretch of imagination. In fact, the data suggested something very different. Now, most scientists, when faced with data that don't fit their hypothesis, will conclude that there is something wrong with the dataset or that the experimental measurements are somehow flawed. Or they will produce a softened variant of the hypothesis, one that does not need to be rejected in the face of the available data after all.

In what we should now begin to recognize as the hallmark of a truly great scientist, Bohman did nothing of the kind. Instead he began to realize that Mother Nature was trying to tell him something he had not anticipated. But he still didn't know how to analyze the data to best address the research questions. He began reading papers on separation experiments, published by a young American psychiatrist who had trained with early leaders in the field of statistical genetics and who seemed to be developing innovative approaches to parsing out the influence of genetic and cultural inheritance. They met at a conference and discussed the possibility of a collaboration. The American immediately realized the value of the Swedish data. In what became the beginning of a lasting collaboration, he came up with a sophisticated statistical approach that enabled the cross-fostering analysis.

In brief, the analysis, which over the years has become an official citation classic, showed that adopted men ran a risk of developing early onset, severe alcoholism that reflected the risk of their biological, not their adoptive, fathers. This confirmed indications from earlier, more limited adoption studies such as that carried out by Donald Goodwin and Sam Guze of Washington University, St. Louis, using a Danish adoption registry.[6] For good measure, Bohman and Sigvardsson replicated their Stockholm Adoption Study fifteen years later, using the adoption registry from the second largest Swedish city, Göteborg. The results were nearly identical.[7] Similar data followed from other groups.

Of course, if this research really is all that important, readers in the United States may wonder why they have not heard of these groundbreaking Swedes. It is a safe bet that neither Bohman nor Sigvardsson is a familiar name to most Americans, not even to those who study addiction. Instead psychiatrists and addiction scientists all over the world are more likely to be familiar with another name, Bob Cloninger, who is one of the most cited psychiatric researchers of all time. The author of some four hundred scientific research papers and a member of the Institute of Medicine of the U.S. National Academy of Sciences, he was for years chair of the psychiatry department at Washington University. Cloninger is the young American with whom Bohman once initiated a collaboration, and with whom he then continued to publish for many years.

Although clearly a landmark, the adoption studies could still be questioned. In some of them, it was not possible to exclude that exposure to the intrauterine environment was a factor, although that could not be the case in the Stockholm Adoption Study, which for that very reason restricted the analysis to fathers and sons. Even with that caveat taken care of, few adoptions occur just outside the delivery room. One could speculate that even a few months at the beginning of life could have a decisive, lasting influence on how people turn out. But the adoption studies marked the beginning of an era in which much improved insights into the role of heritable and environmental factors for addiction risk were achieved. In the more than three decades that have passed since these seminal studies, a much more complete picture has emerged from a range of different approaches. The basic findings of a substantial genetic contribution to the risk for developing addictive disorders have received firm support over these years. The most important source of this expanding knowledge has been twin studies, originating from large twin registries in Denmark, Sweden, Minnesota, and Virginia, and from the Vietnam era twins.

Before going into those findings, I need to say a few words about twin studies. Despite a fascination with twins that occasionally results in newspaper headlines like "They Got Married on the Same Date Without Even Knowing It," the scientific opportunities offered by twin studies are in my experience not well understood by the public. It is not unusual to hear research results originating from twins dismissed with comments such as "of course twins will be similar to each other in their risk for addiction, they grow up in the same families. So any similarities don't have to reflect genetics, at all." In fact, twin studies do not base their assessment of genetic influences on the degree of similarity between twins in general. What they do instead is make clever use of the fact that twins come in two varieties. Fraternal twins are genetically no more similar than any other pair of brothers or sisters—they share, on average, 50 percent of their genes. Identical twins, on the other hand, are just that—identical. All the three billion or so letters in their DNA code are the same. So it really doesn't matter whether, for instance, one twin being alcohol dependent is accompanied by the other sharing the same fate in 10, 40, or 70 percent of cases. What matters is whether that degree of similarity, called concordance, is the same or different in identical and fraternal twins.

If concordance is the same in fraternal and identical twin pairs, despite the much higher degree of genetic similarity within the identical pairs, then genetics simply cannot matter. In that case, heritability, the proportion of risk contributed by genes, must be zero, and any differences between twins must be attributed to environmental influences or chance. But if, on the other hand, the concordance within identical twin pairs is significantly higher than that within fraternal pairs, then genes must contribute, at least if some simple assumptions hold. This is not to say that shared family environment could not still play a role. The beauty of this approach is, however, that the role of the environment does not interfere with our ability to measure the genetic risk. This is because environmental factors presumably affect twins to the same extent whether they are fraternal or identical. Your environment—whether, for instance, your parents were alcoholics themselves—presumably does not care much if the fertilized egg from which you originated happened to split moments after conception, resulting in there essentially being two of you.[8] If this assumption holds true, then whatever the contribution of the environment was, it can be simplified out of the equation.

Applying some sophisticated math—called structural equation modeling—to this kind of data allows an equation consisting of three terms to be estimated. For any trait, such as in our case a diagnosis of an addictive disorder, and for any level of total risk for developing that trait, that risk is decomposed into three components that can be expressed as percentages, obviously adding up to 100:

- a heritable component, or "heritability"
- an environmental component that is shared between children in a family, such as growing up with alcoholic parents, or "shared environment"
- a term that bundles all the different life experiences that are unique to the individual—say, having been in a car accident—including sheer good or bad luck, or "individual environment"

In 2012 Ken Kendler of Virginia Commonwealth University received the Mark Keller Award from the National Institute on Alcohol Abuse and Alcoholism for his pioneering work on the genetics of alcoholism. This work, much of it carried out with his former colleague Carol Prescott, now at the University of Southern California, has used twin data to answer many of the key questions of the field. The award lecture, one of the most enjoyable and thought provoking I have heard in many years, showed what a great rabbi the world lost when Ken decided to become a physician scientist, and what a wonderful scientist and academic teacher we gained in the bargain. Pooling available research from many sources, the different twin studies agree to a remarkable degree on the heritability of alcoholism, which they estimate to be somewhere around 55 percent. The same twin data show that the shared environment also contributes to a significant extent, accounting for just under 40 percent of the risk. The heritability of other addictive disorders has been estimated in the same range, with heritability of addiction to opiates and cocaine perhaps being slightly higher than that to alcohol.[9] This places addictions in a range of genetic influence that is higher than that for depression or anxiety disorders but lower than for schizophrenia, bipolar illness, or autism.

The pooling of the various twin studies yields some other important insights. In contrast to what Bohman and his colleagues thought, heritability of alcoholism seems to be almost identical for men and women. And in a case in which it has been possible to examine whether heritability of alcoholism has changed over half a century of changing societal conditions, little difference over time was in fact found. By the way, these heritability estimates from the twin studies are if anything likely to be underestimates. As Kendler points out, establishing a diagnosis of an addictive disorder such as alcoholism is fraught with uncertainty, and that adds noise to the calculations. If the data are corrected for that uncertainty, the true heritability of alcoholism is likely closer to 70 percent.

By now maybe I have convinced you about the proportion of addiction risk that comes from genes. Or maybe you did not need convincing, in which I case I have perhaps reinforced everything you already knew, hopefully in an interesting way. In either case, it is time to make life a bit harder. Having come this far, how about if I told you that the coveted, hard-earned heritability numbers we have painstakingly gone over perhaps are not meaningless but mean something quite different from what one may first think? To illustrate the fundamental issue at hand, let's carry out a thought experiment. Clearly addictions are in the broad category of complex traits—think, for example, of positive emotionality or mental toughness, both estimated to be about 50 percent heritable[10]—to which both genes and environment contribute, and which are important for how people fare in life. Let's now imagine a dream society in which we have identified every environmental factor that adversely influences these traits, and where we have waved a magic progressive wand to eliminate each of those factors. Likewise, in this society, we have identified every positive environmental influence and made sure that every citizen has equal access to it. These interventions would clearly have a major positive impact overall. But because everyone is now exposed to the same optimal environment, there can no longer be a contribution from the environment to differences in how people turn out. Because everyone is exposed to the same perfect environment, any remaining differences between people, although perhaps smaller than before, must now entirely be caused by genes. With the exception of a small term due to chance, heritability all of a sudden approaches 100 percent.

This extreme example of an ideal society has not been achieved anywhere yet, not even in Sweden. But it illustrates a fundamental aspect of heritability. As a measure of how much influence genes have, it is relative rather than absolute. And any estimate of this measure is valid only under the conditions under which it was obtained. Following this thought, maybe the heritability of some important trait on which people differ is lower in a rough, capitalist society but higher in an affluent, well-educated liberal paradise? If you think I am joking, think again. The sweeping claim is often made that aspects of intelligence are highly heritable. People who don't like that idea dismiss this claim in an equally sweeping manner. But neither statement may be all that meaningful. A remarkable piece of work assessed twins at different levels of socioeconomic status and found that in impoverished families, environmental factors accounted for 60 percent of individual differences, while the contribution of genes was close to zero. In contrast, in affluent families the result was almost exactly the reverse.[11] Another way of saying this is that if a person's material resources are very limited, they put a limit on achievement so far below the person's full, genetically determined potential that those heritable determinants don't matter much. If, on the other hand, a person doesn't have any constraint from material resources, then only biological endowment will set the limit.

To properly interpret the results of research on how much genes contribute to addiction risk, we must thus be careful how we frame them. The message so far can perhaps be stated like this: the contribution of genes to the risk for developing alcoholism and other addictive disorders is somewhere between 55 and 70 percent in mostly white populations of industrialized, Western countries in the past half century. Beyond that, it is anybody's guess. There are no records of good twin studies in the papyrus rolls recovered from ancient Egypt.

Establishing the extent to which addictive disorders are heritable is a major scientific advance and settles issues that are as important as they have been contentious. Yet at the same time, these data do not tell us much that is useful about what characteristics or "traits" people inherit that put them at risk for addiction. The heritability numbers say even less about the specific gene variants that contribute to those characteristics. Answers to those questions are not just of academic interest. Those are the answers that ultimately will be needed if we are to put knowledge about genetics of addiction in the service of patients and their families.

In my experience, physicians, policy makers, and others who are keen to improve public health can talk all they want about the dangers of drinking too much or using drugs. And we do. People nod politely and then go on with their lives. It is only when people are able to relate the data to their own lives—perhaps when they can see parallels to that uncle who didn't fare so well—that the risk feels real, and that the information is able to plant a seed of change. Because of this psychology, it will only be once we are able to make predictions about individual risk that we will be able to make personalized interventions and more effectively prevent harmful outcomes. Those interventions can for starters be of the simplest possible kind, one for which we have already seen an example. We can simply advise people at high genetic risk to abstain from a drug that might otherwise kill them, even though others may be able to use the same substance without much harm and with enjoyment. In the process, this distinction effectively gets us away from a double standard, a moralizing position of talking about how bad alcohol is while allowing it to be marketed and sold.

And beyond prevention there is of course the promise of personalized treatment. Once individual heritable factors behind addiction become better understood, we will finally be able to use advances of genetics to guide development of new medications. We will see in the following that different genetic factors contribute in different cases, and once we are able to identify those factors, we will be able to choose the right medication for a patient. For all this promise to materialize, we will need to know much more about the specific gene variants that are involved, not only on average in the population but also in the individual case. Some progress has been made to advance this type of knowledge, but in general the specific traits and genes that carry addiction risk have turned out to be a lot harder to identify than many of us had hoped.

An important reason is probably that different people, even though they may qualify for the same addiction diagnosis, are in fact very different. One person may quietly increase his alcohol consumption over many years while holding a job and supporting a family, until at the age of fifty or so he can finally no longer be without alcohol and starts planning his life around the drug. In contrast, someone else may start drinking early in life, tolerate excessive amounts of alcohol right away, and become aggressive when drunk, in ways so disruptive that she never succeeds in getting an education or a job. One person may be anxious and drink just so that he can leave his home for the grocery store. Someone else may be impulsive and not give much thought to consequences of consuming excessive amounts of drug for performing adequately at work the following day. To make things even more complicated, people who have a high genetic risk for addiction may not require much environmental influence to develop a diagnosis. But others, even without much genetic vulnerability, will ultimately develop the same diagnosis if they keep using a drug for a long time, to the point that their brains undergo changes described in prior chapters.[12]

In the practice of medicine, we tend to focus on what people who seek treatment have in common so that we can establish a diagnosis and use that diagnosis as a basis for treatment. Addiction medicine is no exception. But while people with an addiction diagnosis may all seem quite similar, they are in fact, in many equally important ways, fundamentally different. A way of thinking about this is that there are many different pathways through which a person can get to the point of qualifying for a clinical diagnosis of an addictive disorder. By the time patients seek treatment, they may be similar in the sense that their lives center around seeking out and consuming alcohol or drug in excessive amounts, at the expense of other aspects of life. That does make it critically important to identify the addictive disorder as a clinical problem that requires attention. But that is just a snapshot, here and now; it does not tell us much about the pathway through which the patient got here. It may therefore entirely miss equally critically important information about what biological and psychological mechanisms have become engaged along the way. To me this is much like a diagnosis of heart failure. Most people are familiar with the symptoms of a patient who receives that diagnosis. The swollen legs and the shortness of breath are characteristic. But that is also an end-stage condition. In one patient it perhaps resulted from coronary disease. In someone else it was caused by hypertension. If you had one of these underlying conditions, you would definitely not want to be treated for the other.

What hints do we have, then, about traits that set people on different pathways to addiction? One important indication comes, once again, from twin studies. When thousands of twin pairs were evaluated for ten of the most common psychiatric and addictive disorders, there was a clear pattern. Judging from their genetics, the disorders seemed to fall into two distinct groups, indicating that the conditions within each group belong together genetically. What that means is that people who have them are likely to share many gene variants that result in risk. But the disorders in each of the groups also seemed to share clinical characteristics. Scientists typically classify the psychiatric disorders within one of these groups as internalizing, and the other as externalizing.[13] These concepts are quite intuitive. In the internalizing group we find conditions in which people seem to turn inward, such as in fear or anxious misery. In this group we find the different types of anxiety disorders as well as major depression.

In the externalizing category are conditions where people instead turn their attention and actions outward. Addictive disorders for the most part fall in this category, together with antisocial personality disorder and conduct disorder. Before we proceed, there is an important caveat to interpreting this finding. Antisocial personality is a rather stigmatizing condition, characterized by a habitual pattern of lying, lawbreaking, and lacking in empathy with other people. Finding addictive disorders in the same group as this condition does not imply that the two are the same. What it means is that genes and traits that put individuals at risk for one of the disorders to some extent also contribute to the risk for developing the other. And among the most prominent traits shared by disorders within the externalizing group are various aspects of impulsivity. Having read in a prior chapter how rash actions, steep temporal discounting, and other aspects of impulsive behavior predispose for compulsive drug use in both people and animal experiments, this should hardly come as a surprise. In short, a major pathway through which genes are likely to put people at risk for addiction seems to be through various impulsive traits. It is easy to see how that might happen. Drugs have powerful reinforcing or rewarding effects in the short term; their adverse consequences are more distal in time. If, for genetic reasons, you are unable to properly gauge the value of short-term outcomes against their long-term cost, your risk of excessive drug use would only be expected to be higher.

Other characteristics are perhaps more surprising. Marc Schuckit at the University of California, San Diego,[14] found some of these by applying an ingenious approach. He recruited several hundred people in their twenties who themselves had not yet developed alcohol problems. Some of them were sons of alcoholics; others did not have any alcoholism in the family. Presumably the former group would carry a genetic susceptibility to developing addiction, while the latter would not. The idea was to carefully examine both groups early enough so that any differences between them would have a better chance of reflecting their preexisting susceptibility without being complicated by alcohol problems of their own. The researchers then planned to follow their subjects over years to see what characteristics observed prior to the onset of alcohol problems predicted the development of alcoholism.

In the end the research group engaged and examined over four hundred research participants. Among those who had alcoholism in the family, there was an interesting characteristic: they did not seem to be very sensitive to alcohol. In particular, they did not seem to be much influenced by the ability of alcohol to result in impaired balance, something that can be measured as increased body sway. Not every son of alcoholics had this characteristic, but it was present among almost half of them. The same was occasionally found in people without a family history as well, but in the latter group only between one in ten and one in twenty people showed the trait. The importance of these findings emerged over the following years. People with the "low response" to alcohol went on to develop alcoholism four times more often than those with a normal level of responding in 56 versus 14 percent of cases, respectively. A simple way of interpreting the data is that people normally have a brake on their alcohol intake. Alcohol activates brain reward systems, but it is not very potent, so quite a bit of intake is required for more pronounced effects. But at those levels of intake, most people also feel quite impaired, and so they respond with an aversion or simply become unable to continue their intake. If, because of genetic factors, this built-in brake is absent, then it makes sense that the risk of progressively increasing consumption and ultimately becoming addicted grows.[15]

There are other traits, too. For instance, people with social anxiety are more likely to develop all kinds of substance use disorders. A clinical diagnosis of social anxiety disorder is only modestly heritable, with genes being responsible for about 30 percent of the risk. But the personality trait central to developing the clinical conditions—fear of being negatively evaluated by others—has a heritability around 50 percent.[16] It is easy to see a pathway that leads to addiction for a person with this trait. For these people, attending every social function is torture; it feeds scary fantasies about what terrible thoughts others may have about them. Even just eating lunch in a diner is a nightmare. In the mind's eye, everyone is watching, just waiting for you to spill ketchup all over your tie, something that makes your hands shake just enough to spill the ketchup all over your tie. If you repeatedly make the experience of these fears go away after taking alcohol as a pretreatment, then of course very powerful learning occurs. This is a classic case of establishing and escalating drug use for its negatively reinforcing properties. But as we have already learned, repeated drug taking will result in neuroadaptations in the brain pathways that control stress and anxiety reactions. This is therefore a path that leads straight to the dark side of addiction. In the absence of drug, the fears will get even worse, and the incentive to resume drug use will become progressively greater.

What we have described here is a very different pathway to addiction than that which starts as an impulsive, externalizing daredevil, walking the handrails of highway overpasses. The genetic risk factors are unlikely to overlap much. Yet the end result, by the time the patient seeks treatment, will satisfy diagnostic criteria for the same disorder, tempting the thought process of the treating physician to apply the same treatment. There are other traits, too, but you get the idea. We need to, as Danielle Dick at Virginia Commonwealth University likes to say, "deconstruct addiction" and find the different component traits that make up both the risk factors and the diagnosis itself.[17] I expect that understanding those component traits will make it easier to identify specific biological mechanisms that contribute to an addiction in the individual case and to target it with treatment appropriate for that particular individual. Many years from now, once we have understood the component traits and the biological mechanisms that drive them, maybe we will be able to reassemble diagnostic categories that make more sense and provide better help for choosing the right treatment. Perhaps those will be something like "impulsive alcoholism," "opioid-reward dependent alcoholism," or "socially anxious alcoholism."

Although I wish this view were my invention, it is of course nothing of the kind. It is merely an application to addictive disorders of a very influential concept proposed in the early 1970s and then reiterated more recently by the behavioral geneticist Irving Gottesman of the University of Minnesota in the context of his research on schizophrenia. To put things in the language of a professional geneticist, a trait—such as having a diagnosis of hypertension or an addictive disorder—is called a phenotype, from the

Greek words *phainein*, "to show," and *typos*, "type." As is often the case, the Greek roots tell us something important about the concept. Because showing is an inherent part of the word, it is clear that the trait should be directly visible or observable. But if things that under the surface are quite different can appear the same way to unaided observation, then we can hope that, beneath the surface, we might be able to find other traits, closer to the biological underpinnings of the disorder, and ultimately the genes that shape the biological risk factors. Gottesman describes these component traits, which he calls endophenotypes, like this:

> Endophenotypes, measurable components unseen by the unaided eye along the pathway between disease and distal genotype, have emerged as an important concept in the study of complex neuropsychiatric diseases. An endophenotype may be neurophysiological, biochemical, endocrinological, neuroanatomical, cognitive, or neuropsychological (including configured self-report data) in nature. Endophenotypes represent simpler clues to genetic underpinnings than the disease syndrome itself, promoting the view that psychiatric diagnoses can be decomposed or deconstructed, which can result in more straightforward—and successful—genetic analysis.[18]

Next we will see what the concept of endophenotypes has to offer for gene findings, and how it helps us understand some of the challenges that have so far prevented much of the promises of molecular genetics of addiction to materialize.

So what about the genes? Scientists are beginning to learn about some genes that contribute to addiction risk, too, and I am now almost ready to talk about them. But before I do, I still need to discuss how genes vary between people, introduce some terms with which that variation is described, and talk about how the influence of a gene variant for the risk of developing a disease can be determined. If this sounds like a crash course on aspects of modern molecular genetics, that is because it is. It is actually not possible to make sense of newspaper headlines such as "Alcoholism Gene Found"[19] without understanding these basics. Though I will only bring in the facts and terms that really matter, even those will be simplified, so I apologize ahead of time to my geneticist friends.

Remember, a gene is, loosely defined, a stretch of DNA string from which a protein is produced. Proteins are stitched together through the workings of cellular machinery by adding, one by one, individual building blocks made up of amino acids. There are twenty of those in nature. In contrast, the DNA code consists of only four letters—T, C, A, and G—and these are used to code what amino acid to add next to the growing protein string, using "words" of three letters each. As the astute reader will quickly realize, this means there are many more code words than there are amino acids. Indeed, as the 1968 Nobel laureates Nirenberg, Khorana, and Holley found, each amino acid has more than one triplet encoding it. This is important because it means that even when we find a mutation that changes the genetic code, that mutation may leave the meaning of the code unaltered. The sequence may still code for the same amino acid, in which case it is called "synonymous," and may not matter at all. This is in contrast to "nonsynonymous," meaning that the protein will actually contain a different amino acid in that position.

Preceding the DNA code that contains the blueprint for which amino acids to put together to make a protein, a gene typically starts with a sequence of code letters that contain "promoter elements." These are places where components of cellular machinery bind and determine, not what the protein that is about to be produced will look like, but rather how much of it will be made. The DNA code for consecutive amino acids then follows but is contained in pieces, or "exons." These are segments of code that are interspersed with "introns," stretches that will not be translated into protein. To send a work order from the DNA blueprint to the protein-building factory of the cell, the DNA code is copied to a messenger RNA (mRNA). The immature form of the work order is a copy of both exons and introns, but before reaching the protein factory, it matures into the final protein-making template by "looping out" and removing the segments of code that correspond to introns, through a process called splicing. The mature mRNA finally has a tail that does not contain any protein-making code but can allow various cellular signals to fine-tune how much protein will ultimately be made.

The point of this crash course is that the proteins are the business end of the genome. They fall into several categories. Some become structural elements of cells or what lies between cells. Others are enzymes that turn over fuels to energy or carry out other cellular functions. A third class make up a slew of signaling molecules, such as hormones or neurotransmitters. Although people vary in their DNA sequence, for this variation to have functional consequences, it has to influence the function of proteins, by changing either their amino acid composition or the amount in which they are made. There are less than thirty thousand genes in the human genome, but because of the opportunities for rearrangement of the building blocks that come from individual exons—alternative splicing—there are many more proteins. There are millions of places in the genome where two different people may have a different code, or be "polymorphic." The simplest case is a replacement of a single DNA code letter for another one, say C → G, called a "single nucleotide polymorphism" (SNP). Other cases may be where a couple of letters have been lost or gained, called insertion-deletion polymorphism. When two people carry gene variants that contain different code letters, they are said to have different alleles of that gene, and the most common way people differ in their genetics is called allelic variation.[20] But remember, allelic variation will not matter much unless it influences the structure or amount of a protein. So what we are after in the end is *functional* variation.

How do we go about trying to find gene variants, or alleles, that contribute risk for addictive disorders? Although this is a monumental task, the basic logic is deceptively simple. Let's say we find an SNP where some people carry a C, while others have a G. Of course we all carry two copies of almost all genes—one from mom, the other from dad—so in reality people can be CC, CG, or GG at this position in the genome. Now let's find one hundred people with a diagnosis of alcoholism and another hundred without it, determine their genotype, and count how many alleles read C in the respective group. Remember, since every individual carries two copies of the gene, there are two hundred alleles in each group. Let's say 152/200, and thus 76 percent of these are C among alcoholics, while only half that, 76/200 or 38 percent, are C among the healthy controls. If one applies some relatively simple statistics to these numbers, it turns out that the probability of this happening by chance is less than 1/10,000. So as true scientists, we reject the null hypothesis that this was a random event. Instead we conclude that we have found an association between this particular gene variant and alcoholism. With only slightly more sophisticated math, we can also calculate what percentage of the risk for alcoholism can be attributed to this variant.

Simple, right? Not really. There are more sources of error for this kind of analysis than there is room in this book. Just to take one issue that is common and has plagued this field, there are obviously systematic differences in DNA sequence between people based on their ancestry. Otherwise our babies would not differ in visible ways! But if C happens to be more common among people of African descent than among Caucasians, and there happen to be more of the former than of the latter in our patient group, we would get a higher allele frequency and a statistical association no matter what disease we looked at. That association would have nothing to do with what we wanted to study, and everything to do with how we had selected our subjects. Many of the early gene findings were simply artifacts of this nature. There are increasingly good ways of correcting for that kind of error. But even once we establish a real, valid association, it does not tell us anything about how this variant contributes to the risk. In fact, because the genome contains so many variants, and because these tend to travel together in packs, glued to one another as chromosomes are transmitted from parents to offspring and occasionally rearranged through a process called recombination, we have no idea if the statistically associated variant is the one that contributes to the differences between patients and controls. It could just as well be another variant that does the job, one that is located some ways up- or downstream of the allele that we have studied within the DNA sequence, and that we did not even know about but that statistically travels together with our C, say, 90 percent of the time.

In the early days of the gene-finding field, scientists would literally count frequencies of one or a few markers in genes they suspected might have something to do with addiction risk, perhaps in regions of the genome identified through a different methodology, called linkage analysis. Several of the earliest gene associations were established using this kind of cumbersome approach, for instance, by the long-running, NIAAA-sponsored Collaborative on the Genetics of Alcoholism (COGA). As technology evolved, however, it became possible to simultaneously determine people's DNA code at a million or even several million SNPs at the same time and carry out what are called whole genome association studies. Once we are able to apply that kind of brute force, surely we must be able to crack which gene variants contribute to addiction risk?

Not really. It is true that there are some findings. The best-established gene associations are with variants of genes from which the body makes enzymes, the little chemical factories that break down alcohol. After it has been ingested and done its job in the brain, alcohol gets broken down, first to the rather nasty chemical acetaldehyde, which normally is not present in the body, and only then to acetate, which the body can use for fuel. Although acetaldehyde makes people feel really sick, this is usually not much of a problem because the rate at which it in turn is converted to acetate is so fast that we don't accumulate much of the toxic intermediary. But about 80 percent of Asians or their descendants have a gene variant that makes them generate acetaldehyde from alcohol about fifty to a hundred times faster than the rest of us. Because this is much faster than the body can convert aldehyde to acetate, the toxic metabolite will now accumulate. In about half these people, this is made even worse by another genetic variant that means that the next step in the reaction, the breakdown of acetaldehyde, is made unusually slow, combining to a particularly pronounced accumulation of the toxic metabolite. These people will react to alcohol intake with a flushing reaction, also called the Asian flush syndrome or Asian glow. Most of them will for that reason experience alcohol as being quite unpleasant. After all, this is the same effect that results from drinking after having taken Antabuse, the very purpose of which is to deter drinking by making alcohol intake intensely unpleasant. It is perhaps unsurprising, then, that people with the gene variants resulting in the flushing reaction have a consistently decreased risk of developing alcoholism. Note that in this case we don't only have an "association"—we have a mechanism.

There is more. In 2004, COGA investigators found an association between alcoholism and a variant of the brain receptor for the neuro-transmitter GABA. This is the receptor through which both alcohol and Valium act to produce their dampening effects, so it clearly seems to be relevant. Most important, the association is real. Other associations had been reported before but often failed to replicate in independent studies. The GABA-receptor finding, in contrast, has been independently replicated several times by now. Yet to this day, while we have an association, we don't quite have a mechanism. The SNPs that show the association are located in introns, and it is so far unclear if they are functional.[21] An even more important advance came in 2007, when a couple of genome-wide associ-ation studies pointed to an association between nicotine addiction and a gene that codes for one of the proteins from which the nicotinic receptor is assembled. That association was then replicated by the Icelandic DECODE group, which uses the entire population of Iceland as a genetic laboratory.[22] The DECODE paper also elegantly showed that the guilty gene variant, as would be expected if it significantly contributes to people's smoking, is also associated with lung cancer and cardiovascular disease. In this case there is a bit more of a mechanism. The SNP that causes the association does lead to a receptor that has altered function, and imaging studies have shown that it alters brain function, by modulating the strength of connection between two components of the brain reward circuitry.[23]

There are other advances, but this should convey the idea. Here is, how-ever, the dilemma. We have previously established that 50–70 percent of addiction risk is caused by genes. Yet if we add up the risk of the most likely hits in whole genome association studies, we can account for, at best, a few percent of the disease risk. But if we are scanning the whole genome, and if genes contribute as much as we know they do, then most of the heritability is missing. The situation is similar for all complex behavioral disorders, as well as complex nonbehavioral conditions such as diabetes. This has been called the missing heritability or, more fancifully, the dark matter of the genome. It has resulted in quite a bit of disappointment after the initial fanfare to celebrate the completion of the Human Genome Project, which raised hopes that we would soon understand the genetic basis of most medical conditions.

Scientists have different takes on the issue. Many hard-core geneticists say that our sample sizes simply are still too small. If we didn't find enough genes in studies that used 10,000 people, then we should use sample sizes of 100,000 instead. Studies of populations this size have in fact been published, often by pooling many different studies carried out in different countries. I am personally not convinced this approach is going to solve the problem we are facing. It is true that with increasing sample sizes, our chances to find associations between gene variants and disease do increase, but we will be finding associations that have smaller and smaller contributions. So I can't see how that is going to address the problem of the missing heritability.

There is a complementary view that uses a different approach. The whole-genome association approach rests on the widely held assumption that common gene variants cause common disorders. For us to find an association, the same common gene variant, or allele, that contributes to risk needs to be present in many of the people who have the disorder. But what if many different, less common variants can all have similar consequences? What if any such unusual variant, not only anywhere in, say, the GABA-receptor gene, but anywhere in one of the many genes that are involved in GABA neurotransmission, can increase alcoholism risk? If that is the case, that is not something we will ever find in a whole-genome association study, at least not the way those are done now.

If many unusual, rather than a few common, gene variants contribute to addiction risk, then other approaches may be better suited to identify the pathways that are involved. Or at least this other approach offers a complementary strategy. To explain it, let me use an example provided by a recent paper from the laboratory of David Goldman at the NIAAA.[24] David's group obtained DNA from one of the most extreme phenotypic groups you can imagine: Finnish men convicted for impulsive murder. The lab sequenced parts of each participant's genome in search of mutations that are rare but have a dramatic effect: they disrupt a gene altogether, creating the human equivalent of a knockout mouse. The Goldman lab found that one such mutation can occur in a gene that codes for a particular serotonin receptor. When mice had the same gene knocked out, they also showed highly impulsive behavior. The human mutation was present only in Finns, so it can't cause impulsivity in other populations. But it confirms that serotonergic function is critical for impulsivity, and it suggests that any mutation in this pathway might influence the risk for impulsive traits, and therefore also for addiction.

Although my own laboratory does a fair amount of genetics, all that work is in the context of pharmacology. I am not a real geneticist. I follow the advances described here with equal amounts of fascination and frustration. In many ways the field has made unbelievable progress. On the horizon is the day when each of us will be able to carry our whole genome sequence, obtained once and for all at a cost of less than $1,000, on a card in our wallets, or perhaps on a chip injected once and for all under the skin. Yet the search for individual gene variants that are mechanistically important for addictive disorders, in a way that would help me as a clinician treat patients, has for the most part been less successful than most of us hoped and expected even a decade ago.

For now it seems that a reasonable position is to be fascinated by genes but to let clinical work be guided by the much more mature knowledge of classical genetics. We know useful things, and we should make a habit of putting those to good use. If a person had a father and a grandfather who were alcoholics, if that person himself or herself appears to have low sensitivity to depressant alcohol effects and perhaps also shows impulsive traits, then it important for that individual to be counseled about the high genetic risk of alcoholism.

If you ask me, taking a good family history is probably more important at the moment than sequencing the patient's genome.

14

MOLECULAR CULPRITS

B Y NOW WE should finally be ready to spend some time talking about drugs themselves. I have outlined much of the brain machinery that addictive substances hook into, and the inherited vulnerabilities that lead to different levels of risk between people. I have also described enough of the behavioral phenomena that result. That allows me to now shift focus and let a few of the molecules that people actually become addicted to take center stage. In doing so, it is my intention to be quite selective. This is not primarily a book about drugs as such—excellent descriptions of those can be found elsewhere.[1] This is first and foremost a book about people, their brains, how they become affected by addiction, and how they can be treated. The study of addictive substances as pharmacological agents is a field that obviously intersects in a major way with those topics, but it has its own perspective and a somewhat different flavor.

However, to fully understand the dynamics of drug addiction, both in populations and in individual people, it is helpful and almost necessary to discuss some real-world prototypes of addictive drugs. Along the way it is worthwhile to consider the history of these substances and how their impact on human lives has evolved over that history. That perspective should help us capture some salient characteristics of the interaction between molecules and brains and allow some themes to emerge. One of those themes is that availability is a major determinant of drug use, and that drug use for that reason spreads in ways that are similar to epidemics of infectious agents. Another theme is that purity and route of administration, trivial though they may sound, are major determinants of addictive potential. That is because the rate with which drug effects hit the brain is a major determinant of the high people experience. As a corollary of that rule, we will see that the long-term changes that usher the switch to the "dark side of addiction" are also most effectively driven when the initial, rewarding hit of drug high is the most intense. A final theme will be that addictive properties of drugs are to varying degrees influenced by characteristics of the individual. Nowhere is that more pronounced than in the case of alcohol. I will discuss some of the reasons for that.

As examples I will use three categories of drugs that most people are familiar with. The first of these, morphine-like substances, or "opioids," are probably the psychoactive drugs whose use goes the furthest back in the history of mankind. As an aside, the history of these substances is much longer than that. Receptors for morphine-like substances were present as early in evolution as the amoeba. Applying morphine to a bath in which these unicellular organisms are swimming around will make them move toward the drug and also alter the cellular processes through which they ingest nutrients, or "eat."[2] Clearly systems that guide approach behaviors in humans build on elements that evolution developed long before our species appeared on the planet. The next drug group, cocaine and amphetamine-like drugs, which despite some important differences we can bundle under the label "psychostimulants," is important because it hooks right into the core of the brain systems thought to mediate approach behaviors and reward. Alcohol, finally, makes up a substance category of its own but is probably able to fill up a catalog of actions more extensive than any other drug category. It is also, for that very reason, the addictive drug where individual differences in drug effects are the greatest.

"Opium" is in many ways a prototype for all other addictive drugs. Its name refers to dried milk of the opium poppy, *Papaver somniferum*.[3] Opiates are the naturally occurring substances that can be extracted from opium, with morphine being the most important among them. In modern times a number of manufactured opioids, literally meaning "opium-like" substances in Greek, have been added to the formulary. For instance, a painkiller such as fentanyl is entirely man-made but acts in ways that are in principle at least the same as morphine. These drugs are therefore appropriately called opioids. To the human brain, it really doesn't matter if a molecule happened to be extracted from a plant or was made in a laboratory before it hits the brain receptors. And sometimes it is not even possible to know whether it was one or the other—the painkiller codeine, for instance, can either be extracted from the opium poppy or be made in a chemistry lab. Out of deference to proper nomenclature, I will keep using both terms, "opiate" and "opioid," and try to be as precise as possible. But from a clinical perspective, we could just as well go with the broader term "opioids" for all drugs that act in ways similar to morphine. This broader label also covers opiate-like substances, or endogenous opioids, that are made by our own brains and that were discussed in a prior chapter.

Inscriptions on clay tablets tell us that the opium poppy was grown as early as 5,500 years ago by the Sumerians of Mesopotamia, the "land between the rivers" that was the cradle of Western civilization. The Sumerians called their poppy the joy plant, so they must have been aware of its psychotropic properties. From here it took the plant some 2,000 years to reach Egypt. The people of Thebes, the Egyptian capital at the time, became the first large-scale commercial opium growers, giving the plant the name "opium thebaicum." This name still echoes through the millennia in thebain, a constituent of opium poppy from which the common painkiller oxycodone can be made. Seafaring Phoenician and Cretan merchants then brought the desirable opium plant from Egypt to ancient Greece, from where it spread to the rest of Europe and, carried by Alexander the Great's armies, to Persia and India. Ironically, although today associated with the Far East, opium did not arrive in China until the fifth century A.D. Only a few centuries later, however, it was so strongly associated with "Eastern magic" that it was condemned by the Catholic Church, and the Inquisition made sure that its use fell out of fashion in Europe. When opium returned to the West in the sixteenth century, it was as a medicine to suppress pain, called laudanum.

Originally opium was dried and eaten. Taken in this manner, much of the active ingredient is broken down in the gut. Perhaps even more important, taking opium this way makes for a rather slow uptake of what active ingredient remains. Since the high from a drug is related both to the amount of drug that reaches the brain and the speed with which it does so, the slow uptake of opiates taken by mouth limited their addictive potential. Then, in the sixteenth century, Portuguese marine merchants sailing off the cost of China figured out that opium could be mixed with tobacco and smoked. All of a sudden, uptake into the brain was nearly complete and almost instantaneous—truly a "high." Used this way, the drug offered intense rewarding effects that quickly took control of the people using it. The Chinese, with their Confucian culture valuing self-control, considered this practice barbaric. But over the next two centuries, the Portuguese, British, and Dutch all used their colonial powers to promote trade of opium grown in India with the Chinese mainland. The consequences were so disastrous that three Chinese emperors attempted to outlaw the use of opium in the eighteenth century. But the trade was too profitable for the British Empire to give up. Instead the Opium Wars secured the rights for the East India Company to continue the trade, resulting in the misery of opium dens reaching epidemic proportions. To this day the growth of opium in the Golden Triangle (Burma, Thailand, Laos, and Vietnam) is a gift to our times from the colonialism of the British Empire. About a century later the other major opium plantation of the world, the Golden Crescent that spans much of Afghanistan and northern Pakistan, is a product of another great empire and its conquests, that of the late Soviet Union.

In 1803 or possibly 1804, the German pharmacist Friedrich Sertuerner mixed opium with an acid and then neutralized the mix with ammonia. Through this procedure he became the first person on record to extract in pure form the active ingredient of the opium poppy or, for that matter, of any medicinal plant. *Principium somniferum*, or morphine,[4] had arrived. Physicians were somehow convinced that the substance could now finally be used in a precisely controlled and therefore safe fashion. In the late 1820s E. Merck of Darmstadt, Germany, started large-scale commercial manufacturing of the new miracle medicine. In 1843 it was discovered that the effects of morphine were both more immediate and more potent if the drug was injected, increasing its utility in controlling severe pain. The American Civil War saw a great breakthrough for the hypodermic needle as a technology, and its use allowed effective morphine delivery to the massive numbers of wounded soldiers. The rapid pain-relieving actions must have seemed a blessing. But it was soon clear that what had been viewed as a major medical advance was turning into a disaster. After the war large numbers of demobilized soldiers were unable to wean themselves off morphine. By the end of the nineteenth century, there were a quarter million morphine addicts in the United States.

A search for remedies was on. In 1897 Heinrich Dreser, who headed up the pharmacology laboratories of Bayer Industries in Germany, found that a simple chemical modification turned morphine into a drug called diacetylmorphine. Today this chemical is of course better known by the trade name given to it by Bayer on commercially launching it in a cough syrup—"Heroin."[5] The new miracle drug was promoted for many ills. With tuberculosis rampant and no antibiotics yet available to treat pneumonia, the ability of heroin to suppress cough was heaven sent. It was also a more potent analgesic than morphine. Its ability to stop diarrhea was useful, too. But the most important application was thought to be as a cure for morphine addiction. This time, however, it did not take long before the addictive potential of the proposed "cure" itself was realized. Bayer's new wonder drug had an unusually short career. Its provision without a prescription was stopped in the United States in 1913, and all medical use was outlawed in 1919.

Today morphine remains the prototypical medical opiate, while heroin is the prototypical addictive member of the class. There are of course many other opiates and opioids—too many to be discussed here. When teaching these things, my approach is always to first help people understand one or two prototypical drugs in a class, the profile of their actions, and the mechanism through which these actions are produced. This provides a mental structure from which to start. After that, other, related substances can more easily be understood as variations on the theme. For instance, oxycodone is much like morphine but is a bit less potent and is more reliably absorbed when taken by mouth, lasting a bit longer and not causing itching. Fentanyl, on the other hand, once again is similar in its actions to morphine but is much more potent and extremely fast acting. And heroin really *is* morphine as far as the brain is concerned. The small chemical tweak introduced by Wright and Dreser just speeds up its entry into the brain. The chemical additions are then cut off by the body, and the brain is left with morphine that is now free to do its job. So in a way, the development of heroin was just another step in a progression, from slowly raising opiate concentrations in the brain by eating opium, through a faster uptake achieved by smoking opium or injecting morphine, to the ultimate hit—so far—achieved either by vaporizing and inhaling brown heroin or injecting the fully purified, white product. Either of the latter ways leads to an intense hit of euphoria.

Or, I should say, *may* lead to an intense hit of euphoria. Right here we can see how drug effects are a true interaction between the molecules and the brains they hit. Not everybody is prone to euphoria from opiates or opioids. In fact, the people who do respond with pleasurable effects to these drugs are probably a minority. For instance, large numbers of people receive morphine for postoperative pain. If asked, only a few of those report pleasurable effects. Brought up with the commanding, objective, and seemingly unequivocal dose-response curves of my pharmacology training, for years I did not know what to think of this variation. Maybe people were just embarrassed to reveal those pleasurable effects of morphine? That, for many reasons, turns out not to be an explanation. Maybe it simply had something to do with the setting in which opiates were given? There was in those days a widely held perception, since then long shattered by the recent epidemic of prescription opioid abuse, that when opioids are given in a medical setting, the addictive potential just isn't there. It didn't sound unreasonable at the time—after all, environment does matter. Maybe this was just an illustration of that fact?

Then, after having practiced and taught addiction medicine for some fifteen years, having written a textbook for medical students on the topic, and having begun to think that I knew a thing or two, I had my first surgery myself. My colleague Jan-Erik Juto of the Karolinska Hospital, a quiet, highly respected ENT surgery virtuoso, was simply wonderful. But boy, was I in pain after he had messed around inside my face. As I woke up and was wheeled back to the ward, I kept getting morphine. There was some bleeding, too. Nevertheless, around 8 P.M. I rang the bell. When the charge nurse came, her face expressing concern about my well-being, I asked if I could please sneak down to my office, just two floors down in the hospital, and check on some work. She looked at me in disbelief, shook her head, and gave me a lecture on postoperative complications. I let her finish the speech, waited half an hour until the shifts had their handoff at the nurse's station, then quietly left, still in my hospital gown. Once I got to my office, I was able to quickly finish up a paper that at the time seemed important. As I came to my senses the next day, I was equally embarrassed, awestruck, and frightened. The simple fact was, I had probably never felt that good in my whole life. I recall telling my wife about the experience after coming home. She tried to listen, but it was clear that she just didn't understand. After a couple of cesarean sections, morphine to her was just good pain suppression, obtained at the cost of unpleasant nausea. Individual differences in drug responses are, to a large extent, about just that—the individuals involved. And the most permanent ways in which we as individuals differ are of course in our genetics. Personalized medicine is rearing its head, sometimes ugly, sometimes beautiful, almost everywhere we look.

For people who end up taking opiates or opioids for their addictive properties, there is typically a set sequence of events that follow after taking drug. After injecting or inhaling heroin comes a brief rush, an intense feeling of intoxication that lasts only a few minutes and is accompanied by a visceral feeling commonly described by patients as similar to that of an orgasm. This is followed by a high of quiet euphoria that lasts perhaps half an hour. After that, people feel "straight" for a few hours and can seem quite unaffected. But then withdrawal symptoms kick in, and the person starts feeling sick. Other actions of heroin and morphine affect people in a more consistent fashion than the high. Perhaps most important is a triad of effects. First, there is of course a prominent suppression of pain. Second, and perhaps less widely known, secretion decreases or stops from all kinds of glands in the body, such as tear and sweat glands, and the water-excreting glands that line the gut. Third, the centers in the brain stem that provide the pacemaker signals for breathing are suppressed, ultimately resulting in death if respiration is not maintained by some external force.

As already mentioned, only a minority of people experience a high from opioids. We don't yet know exactly why that is, but there is a hint that this is determined by our genes. That hint is provided from another opioid effect, the suppression of pain. People differ in how effectively morphine does that, and those individual differences have been clearly tied to genetics of the mu-opioid receptor gene. We will examine those differences and some of their consequences when we come back to the potential of the opioid antagonist naltrexone as an addiction treatment.

A unique feature of opiates and opioids is that unusually high and rapid tolerance develops both for the high they give rise to and for their other actions. It is actually still not exactly clear how that happens in the brain, either. My textbook in medical school once had all the answers to this, but it has been downhill ever since. From a clinical perspective, however, the high degree of tolerance that develops means that with continued use, people will need to drastically increase their doses just to maintain a certain effect. When they stop using, tolerance typically wears off within about a week.[6] While tolerance wears off, there will in the absence of treatment be a constellation of much feared and unpleasant withdrawal symptoms. These are best thought of as the opposite of the drug effects, so you should know by now what to expect. In a mirror image of the high, mood will be depressed. Analgesia will turn into a flu-like ache throughout the body and goose pimples all over the skin. All glands will start secreting fluid, so that eyes will tear, noses will run, and guts will discharge. Actually, as unpleasant as it is to go "cold turkey" like this, it is with rare exceptions entirely without risk, which is more than can be said about withdrawal from the much less feared drug alcohol.[7] But as cycles of intoxication and withdrawal are repeated, there is with opiates a very powerful allostatic shift, of the kind described in a prior chapter. This syndrome is usually present in fully developed form about two years into heavy use. The patient moves to the dark side of addiction. In the absence of drug, mood now remains low long beyond acute withdrawal, and reactions to stress remain high. This creates a powerful incentive for resumption of drug taking, signaled by cravings that are perhaps more powerful than for any other class of addictive substances. Somehow these cravings often persist for decades and can even be experienced in dreams.

Treatment of opioid withdrawal is commonly called detoxification. Although often thought to require highly specialized skills, it is actually very simple, at least in principle. Tapered doses of almost any opioid given over about five to seven days will allow tolerance to wear off without too much pain. A lot of treatment resources and efforts are devoted to detox. It may seem good to reduce the discomfort of a suffering patient and hope for that also to be a first step toward a drug-free life. But as we will see in a coming chapter, unless given effective treatments such as methadone or buprenorphine maintenance, about 90 percent of heroin addicts will relapse within a year. And when they relapse, having rid themselves of their tolerance is not necessarily a good thing. Out of old habit, patients will frequently go back to taking heroin at doses they were used to before entering detox. The difference is that now, with tolerance gone, those doses are enough to kill them, by shutting off respiration in an overdose. As an example, in the first couple of weeks after leaving prison, where they are typically forced to detox, heroin addicts have an up to eightfold increased risk of dying from an overdose.[8]

This brings us to a final point. Heroin dependence is the deadliest of addictions. At any given time, a heroin addict runs a twenty to fifty times higher risk of dying than a normal, healthy person of the same sex and age. The corresponding number for alcohol is about fivefold. People with heroin addiction die when they stop breathing following an overdose, but also through infections they get by sharing needles, such as bacterial growth on the heart valves, HIV, or hepatitis B and C. There is also a lot of "violent death." All in all, nowhere is the need to provide treatment as much a matter of life and death as in the case of heroin addiction.

"The Divine Plant of the Incas," *Erythroxylon coca*, grows as a bush or a small tree on the slopes of the Andes in present-day Peru, Chile, Colombia, and Bolivia. Its use by early humans of South America is not documented in writing the way we find a written record of early opium use. But radiocarbon dating of archeological findings provides evidence of human coca leaf use and primitive extraction of their contents in this region as early as about eight thousand years ago. By the sixth century A.D., pottery frequently depicted people chewing coca, and supplies of coca leaves were buried together with mummified bodies. At the peak of the Inca Empire, in the fifteenth century A.D., the coca bush was considered to be divine in origin, and growing it was subject to a monopoly restricted to the state and the aristocracy.

After the conquest of the Inca Empire by Francisco Pizarro in 1535, the first references to the coca bush started appearing in print in Spain around 1570. These accounts described how Inca "runners" chewed the coca leaves, mixed up with the alkaline ashes of another plant, to release the active ingredient on long, harsh journeys across the mountain ranges. From the leaves, the runners got the endurance needed for their long, steep climbs and the feeling of satiety that allowed them to travel with only a minimum of food. Later the new European masters would find these same effects useful to extract the most effort possible from their indigenous workers. A Dr. Poeppig reported the following in his 1835 report from journeys in Chile:

> The miner will perform, for twelve long hours, the formidably heavy work of the mine, and, sometimes, even doubles that period, without taking any further sustenance than a handful of parched maize, but every three hours he makes a pause for the purpose of chewing Coca. . . . The same holds good with the Indian, who, as a porter, messenger, or vender of his own productions, traverses the Andes on foot. Merely chewing Coca from time to time, he travels with a load weighing one hundredweight, on his back, over indescribably rough roads and accomplishes frequently ten leagues in eight hours.[9]

But in addition to endurance and satiety, chewing coca leaves was known to give a euphoric pleasure. The Incas used them to celebrate holidays because of these uplifting properties. In fact, the leaves were thought to have powers so magical that they were considered a divine gift, as expressed in this prayer:

> Oh, mighty lord, son of the Sun and of the Incas, thy fathers, thou who knoweth of the bounties which have been granted thy people, let me recall the blessings of the divine Coca which thy privileged subjects are

permitted to enjoy through thy progenitors, the sun, the moon, the earth, and the boundless hills.[10]

Right here are captured some of the key facts worth noting. First, it is clear that the active ingredient of coca leaves acts to stimulate the person, counteracting feelings of fatigue, eliminating hunger, and producing an elevation of mood. This justifies the name psychostimulant. Second, in a parallel to early use of opium, the content of active ingredient in the leaves is relatively low—in the case of coca, on average perhaps only around 1 percent. Its absorption when the leaves are chewed is also rather slow. Under these conditions the addictive potential appears to be more limited than will be observed later in history. Today's crack users would hardly be able to hold a job that involves carrying weights of about 50 kilograms over distances of 50 kilometers a day.

Although coca was imported to Europe shortly after the Spanish conquest of the Inca Empire, it did not become popular until the middle of the nineteenth century. At that time the Italian neurologist Paulo Montegazza experimented with coca after returning home from travels in South America. Based largely on his personal experience, he published a paper in 1859 that would become highly influential. It was entitled "On the Hygienic and Medicinal Properties of Coca and on Nervous Nourishment in General" and gave Montegazza's account of his experience with effects of coca leaves on cognition:

I sneered at the poor mortals condemned to live in this valley of tears while I, carried on the wings of two leaves of coca, went flying through the spaces of 77,438 words, each more splendid than the one before. . . . An hour later, I was sufficiently calm to write these words in a steady hand: God is unjust because he made man incapable of sustaining the effect of coca all lifelong. I would rather have a life span of ten years with coca than one of 10 000 000 000 000 000 000 000 centuries without coca.[11]

By the time Montegazza's paper was published, the method for extracting chemically pure constituents from medicinal herbs that had been developed by Sertuerner had been around for over fifty years and was well known among chemists. With an endorsement like that provided by Montegazza, the extraction method was quickly applied to coca leaves. The same year Montegazza's paper was published, the German chemist Albert Niemann, working out of the University of Göttingen, became the first person to isolate the main active ingredient of coca and named it cocaine. It did not take long before the new miracle drug was mixed into all kinds of tonics, elixirs, and patent medicines. But there was also a simpler, if somewhat less effective, way to extract cocaine. If coca leaves were mixed with alcohol and left for a time, much of the cocaine was eluted into the fluid, and the leaves themselves could be discarded. Among several coca wines produced in this manner, Vin Mariani, a red Bordeaux, became the most successful. It contained about 250 mg of cocaine per liter, was awarded a gold medal by the Vatican, and was happily consumed by the royals of the time. It also inspired a Civil War veteran, John Pemberton of Atlanta, to create his own competing recipe in 1885. His Pemberton's French Wine Coca was initially a success, but shortly thereafter Atlanta and the surrounding county outlawed alcohol. Faced with the need to adapt to the new market, Pemberton replaced his original recipe with one that was free of alcohol. Instead, it was sweetened and carbonated. It was promoted as a cure for many ills, including the morphine addiction suffered by countless veterans of the Civil War, including Pemberton himself. Its name was Coca-Cola. It would contain cocaine until shortly after the turn of the century. To this day it contains an extract of coca leaves, but now with the cocaine removed.

At this point it is tempting to quip about characteristic differences between Europe and the United States. Around the time Pemberton was making money off the coca leaf extract, a Viennese physician was writing to his future wife, expressing hopes that writing learned papers about cocaine would bring him academic recognition. Instead he ended up building an influential school of psychology while high on the drug. That, however, is a story better told by others.[12] From our perspective, what followed is more important. By the first decades of the twentieth century, the addictive potential of cocaine was widely recognized, and its use outlawed almost everywhere outside of South America. Over the following decades there were recurring flare-ups of illicit cocaine use. But during this time the drug was used as the cocaine salt. In this form it has to be insufflated, that is, "snorted" or "sniffled." The efficiency and rate of cocaine uptake are certainly greater when snorting cocaine powder than is possible to achieve by chewing coca leaves. But they are still quite limited. This kind of use is expensive and for the most part is confined to economic and artistic elites. Under these conditions, most users are able to control their use and ultimately discontinue it.

If, however, the cocaine salt is reacted with ammonium bicarbonate or otherwise made to form the free base, it is possible to vaporize it and inhale it through the lungs, something that cannot be done with the salt. This gets the drug into the bloodstream as fast as an intravenous injection. After that, transport into the brain is almost instantaneous. Cocaine has a somewhat unusual chemistry, which helps it get through the barrier into which the brain is wrapped with an unusually high speed. By now the pattern should be familiar. With the almost complete and near instantaneous uptake after the vapor is inhaled, the high reaches unprecedented levels. Along with it, so does the addictive potential. In 1984 a crude formulation of cocaine base hit the streets of American cities on a large scale. Because of impurities, it made a crackling sound as it was vaporized and inhaled. Imitating that sound, the name "crack" was born. With it came the well-known epidemic that ravished entire inner cities. What had been a recreational drug of elites became the curse of poor black communities. Over the coming years, a generation of "crack babies" was born, many of them with irreparable developmental defects from intrauterine cocaine exposure.

Cocaine targets the very core of the brain's reward and approach circuitry. As discussed in a prior chapter, mesolimbic dopamine nerve cells can be thought of as a final common pathway whose activation energizes approach behavior. After dopamine is released from these nerve cells and has transmitted its signal, it is for the most part sucked back into the cells that released it. If you think about it, removing dopamine that has been released from the synapse is a necessity. After you've sent a signal, you must somehow make sure that the signal also comes to an end. How else would you be able to send the next one? You can only send Morse code if the longs and shorts come to distinct stops. The clearance of dopamine is that stop. It is accomplished by a molecular pump that is present in the nerve endings of dopamine cells. Called the dopamine transporter, this protein sits embedded in the nerve ending. It catches a dopamine molecule on the outside of the cell, makes a flip worthy of a freestyle swimmer, and is all of a sudden able to let go of its molecular cargo on the inside. Then it flips back and is ready for the next one. The existence of the transporter was established long before the era of gene cloning. It was well known, for instance, that if you made a soup of nerve endings in the lab and added to it dopamine with a radioactive label on it, the labeled dopamine would quickly be sucked into the nerve endings. An important role of the transporter for the addictive properties of cocaine was also suspected at least since the 1980s. But cocaine binds to more than one place in the brain. For a long time it was not completely clear which effect was most important.

The critical role of the dopamine transporter for psychostimulant properties of cocaine as well as amphetamine was nailed down only in 1996. In the beginnings of the 1990s Susan Amara, then at Yale University, had cloned the dopamine transporter. That allowed Marc Caron and his trainee Bruno Giros at Duke University to make a mouse that was genetically modified and lacked the transporter gene.[13] I still remember my feeling of awe during the poster presentation at the Society for Neuroscience meeting that year. Posters usually show bar graphs, curves, tables. In the crowded halls of a meeting that already in those days attracted close to twenty thousand people, it usually took an effort to concentrate on the figures. This one had them, too, but I actually don't remember any of them. What I do remember is that once I got through the crowd, I saw the little television monitor that Giros had brought with him. It was showing a video of a mouse, filmed while moving freely around in a box, without any drug treatment. It was constantly running around in a way otherwise seen only after a high cocaine or amphetamine dose. Giving those mice cocaine or amphetamine didn't make any difference. I remember thinking, "Missing one gene did all that." I thought of the many people I had met through the years who had always managed to sound wise by saying, "It can't be that simple." Well, I told myself, sometimes maybe it can.

But I get carried away, which easily happens with science that is this exciting. I'm giving you the story backward. Caron and Giros's mouse confirmed beyond reasonable doubt what pharmacologists had long suspected. Cocaine does to the mouse or the human who takes it the same thing that happens when the dopamine transporter gene is knocked out. The drug binds to the transporter and prevents it from sucking back dopamine out of the synapse after it has done its job to transmit the signal. The result is that excessive amounts of dopamine build up in the synapse. With each pulse of dopamine release, the signal onto dopamine receptors is magnified. To a lesser extent, cocaine also blocks similar molecular pumps that exist for the transmitters serotonin and noradrenalin. But it is the elevation of dopamine levels that is behind the addictive potential both in animals and in humans.

Maybe because cocaine acts so directly on a core element of reward and approach circuitry, the high it produces is much more uniform than that from heroin or morphine. There are other important differences, too. Some of the clinically important differences are among consequences of increasing the doses people take. For starters, there are all the psychostimulant effects I have described—a high, increased movement, and so on. But as doses are increased further, the movement effects change in flavor. Rather than running around enthusiastic about everything, people will be locked into stereotypic movements that get repeated over and over again. This is even more pronounced with chronic amphetamine use, where it has earned a specific name: "punding." As doses are increased further still, people become psychotic. In a strictly psychiatric sense, this means that they lose touch with reality and start having delusions, hallucinations, or both. In fact, because of that, dopamine overactivity was long thought to be important for schizophrenia. That turns out to be complicated, however, and the similarities may well be more superficial than we thought. Meanwhile, however, the delusions that come with the use of high psychostimulant doses have a particular flavor. Often they are what a psychiatrist would call persecutory: the patient is convinced that someone is out to get him or her.[14] Of course, with this patient group, it is not always easy to know if this is just a delusion. Just because someone is paranoid does not mean no one is out to get him or her. Another psychotic symptom is a characteristic hallucinatory perception of insects crawling under the skin, the "cocaine bugs" that can make a patient rip through the skin of the forearms to get out the insects. The name is not the best one, since these hallucinations are not unique to cocaine; they are equally common with other psychostimulants, such as methamphetamine.

It was once written in medical textbooks that there is no withdrawal syndrome when people stop taking psychostimulants. In those days the concept of withdrawal was to a large extent shaped by what we knew about opiates and alcohol. The focus was on bodily symptoms—the shakes, running fluids, and aches of the withdrawing morphine or heroin addict, or the tremors, seizures, and delirium of the alcoholic. There is none of that after stopping heavy cocaine use. There is no increase in heart rate or blood pressure either. There is, in fact, not much that can be objectively measured, or heard with the stethoscope. But an important lesson we have learned since those early days is that the really important elements of withdrawal are psychological. And with psychostimulants, just like with other drugs, these follow the opponent process rule. Each binge cycle activates opponent processes that promote low mood. This pushes the patient toward the dark side of addiction. After a binge and its repeated highs, there is a crash. During that withdrawal period, the lingering activity of the opponent processes will increasingly result in symptoms that are opposite to those experienced when using the drug. Perhaps most important when it comes to psychostimulants, the high of intoxication will be followed by an increasingly depressed mood. At times people will be suicidal during this phase. Other withdrawal phenomena follow a similar pattern. The suppressed appetite rebounds, and people eat to catch up the deficits they have accumulated. After staying awake for days during the binge, they sleep a lot. But most important, they shift their affective baseline. In the absence of drug, there is misery. A new cycle is waiting to begin.

Fast forward to present time, and the number of cocaine users has dropped to half of what it was at the height of the epidemic. To some extent cocaine use has been replaced by an increased use of other psychostimulants, perhaps most important methamphetamine, or "meth." If cocaine was a drug of the cities, many of the meth-kitchens are found in rural regions such as Appalachia and Missouri. Many other differences exist. Although I could write a whole chapter about amphetamines, the information about cocaine has provided a solid foundation and a mental structure into which it is relatively easy to insert these drugs. The drugs also affect the dopamine transporter in ways that result in synapses being flooded by excessive accumulation of dopamine. In the case of amphetamines, the transporter is not only blocked; instead these drugs have the ability to turn the pump molecule inside out and get it to pump dopamine *out* of the cell. A body of neuroscience has identified additional differences between the molecular and cellular effects of cocaine and the other psychostimulants. Maybe some of these differences will one day turn out to be very important. For now, however, understanding cocaine as the prototype psychostimulant and then learning a few of the key distinguishing characteristics of the other members in this class goes a long way. The effects of amphetamine are a lot like those of cocaine, although amphetamine does not get into the brain quite as fast. It is, on the other hand, more potent and longer lasting. Methamphetamine, in turn, is much like amphetamine except that it gets into the brain faster. Both are easier to make and cheaper than cocaine.

Psychostimulant addiction is an area of tremendous unmet medical needs. Right now not much in the way of treatment has any convincing scientific data to support its efficacy.

After all the years in my field, I still keep getting in trouble with the word "alcohol." Alcohols really are a whole group of chemicals. The active ingredient in alcoholic drinks is one very specific member of the group—ethyl alcohol, or ethanol, for short. Other alcohols are present in our everyday lives as well, so the distinction is not purely academic. Methanol and butanol, for instance, are often used as fuels or solvents. The sugar alcohol xylitol is used in the food-processing industry and can be found in sugar-free chewing gum. When discussing the drug used and abused by humans, it would therefore perhaps be best to consistently use the proper term, "ethanol." But then again, for consistency, would we perhaps have to say "ethanolism" instead of alcoholism? I am not sure anyone is ready for that. So I will stick with "alcohol," though unless I say otherwise, what I refer to by that name really is ethanol.

Humans have known how to make alcohol for quite some time. It is generally held that our species settled down and embarked on the transition from hunter-gatherers to cultivating the soil some ten thousand years ago. After that it still took a while to figure out how to use yeast to ferment sugars obtained from the crops. But already about six thousand years ago, hieroglyphic inscriptions from ancient Egypt describe production and consumption of wine. Recipes for making wine or beer are also found on clay tablets from Mesopotamia, dated about a millennium later. In ancient Greece, fermented honey—mead—seems to have been the original alcoholic beverage, but wine-producing skills reached Greece about 2000 B.C. Alcoholic beverages were in those days not necessarily consumed only, or even primarily, for their taste or intoxicating properties. Fermented beverages provided a certain degree of protection against growth of bacteria, such as cholera, in drinking supplies. Because of this, fluid consumption in areas where freshwater was not readily available could to a large extent consist of beer or wine. Likewise, when ships went to sea, drinking supplies brought onboard were often not in the form of water but rather as beer. The alcohol content of these beverages was typically relatively low, probably not exceeding 4 percent, so the protection against growth of bacteria was not great—alcohol is best at killing bacteria at concentrations around 70 percent. But I guess a little was better than nothing.

Fermented beverages typically cannot reach an alcohol content beyond 15 percent or so. At higher concentrations the yeast that make the alcohol from sugar poison themselves and die, or at least become unable to keep up production. As already discussed, the rate with which the concentration of a drug rises in the brain is important for the intensity of the high, and therefore for the addictive potential of the drug. It requires quite a bit of determination to quickly work up high blood alcohol concentrations using beverages with low alcohol content. Producing beverages with higher alcohol concentrations became possible only once people learned to make distilled spirits. There are historical accounts of small-scale distillation from ancient Babylonia and Egypt, but successful distillation of quantities useful for human consumption was only achieved by Arab chemists around A.D. 800–900. By the thirteenth century this expertise had spread to Europe.

By the fourteenth century the use of distilled spirits as medicinal elixirs was widespread, for instance, to provide protection or cure from the Black Death. Somewhat ironically, today the number one vodka brand in Iceland *is* Black Death. I guess the name may still be appropriate given the mortality caused by alcohol.

Alcohol is unique among addictive drugs in the way it produces its brain actions. Understanding that basic difference helps to explain why actions of alcohol are more complex and vary between people more than effects of most other addictive drugs. In contrast to heroin or cocaine, alcohol does not have a unique molecular target in the nervous system. It does not bind to, and activate or block, any specific neurotransmitter receptor or transporter. It was once thought that the actions of alcohol on the brain were caused through effects on the sheets of fat that make up the outer membranes of all nerve cells. As an organic solvent, alcohol was in those days thought to become dissolved in those membranes and change their properties. Because neurotransmitter receptors and other signaling molecules are embedded in the cell membranes, changes in membrane properties were somehow thought to change the communication between nerve cells. That does not seem to be the way it works, however. In fact, it is still not entirely clear what the very first steps are in the actions of alcohol. One possibility that is supported by good data is that alcohol enters pockets found in a large family of very important proteins. A prototype for these, called LUSH, is found in the fruit fly, which uses it to recognize certain odors.

Two of the most fundamental transmitter systems of the brain rely for much of their function on receptor proteins that are distal relatives of LUSH and have similar pockets. These systems use for their signals the molecules glutamate and gamma-amino butyric acid, or GABA for short. Each of them has multiple receptors. Within each receptor group, some members send their signal into the receiving cell through a type of mechanism that is different from that described for dopamine or endorphins. The receptors that trigger the most immediate consequences of a glutamate or GABA signal work as molecular channels that are controlled by their respective transmitter. They run from the outside to the inside of the fat sheets that surround the nerve cell. When no transmitter signal has been received, the channels are closed. When the signal arrives, they briefly open. When open, however, these channels are picky about what they let through. In the case of glutamate receptors, they will let through sodium or calcium. In the case of GABA receptors, passage will instead be provided to chloride. In the first case, the result is that the nerve cell will become activated. Chances are it will start firing away, sending signals to other nerve cells. In neuroscience this is referred to as becoming excited, and glutamate is simply the number one "excitatory" transmitter of the brain. When a GABA signal is received and chloride ions are allowed passage into the cell, the result is just the opposite. The activity of the nerve cell that received the signal will be dampened, and the cell will also be less likely to respond to a signal from other nerve cells. GABA is thus the most important inhibitory transmitter of the brain.

When alcohol is taken, the "first hit" is a set of actions on glutamate and GABA systems. In the short term, alcohol intake dials down glutamatergic communication. With alcohol onboard, less glutamate comes out from nerve cells that normally send out this signal, and the response by the neurons that receive it is also smaller for each signal that is received. Since the job of glutamate signals is to activate nerve cells, this set of actions is one way by which alcohol broadly dampens brain activity. But alcohol also strengthens GABA signals, by allowing more chloride to flow into cells that receive them,[15] and probably also by increasing the amount of GABA that is being sent out. Knowing that GABA is the major dampening nerve transmitter of the nervous system, we should expect these actions to contribute to the broad dampening of brain activity produced by alcohol. Together these are indeed the mechanisms through which alcohol is a general brain depressant. The end result is that if alcohol is taken in limited quantities, it will lead to dampening of anxiety, which is all about being excited in the wrong brain areas. At higher levels the depressant actions will also lead to impairment of movement, balance, and thinking. Through the same broadly dampening mechanisms, consumption of higher amounts still will induce sleep, unconsciousness, and ultimately death. As discussed, people vary in their sensitivity to the nervous system dampening actions of alcohol, and this variation is to a large extent genetic. More on that in a bit.

Because glutamate and GABA systems are so fundamental for the millisecond-to-millisecond communication between nerve cells throughout the brain, the first hit of alcohol on these primary targets results in an unusually broad range of secondary effects. Among those are actions on systems we are already familiar with, because we have encountered them as key players in reward from addictive drugs. Perhaps most important among these are the dopamine and endorphin systems. Alcohol intake leads to release of both endorphins and dopamine. These secondary hits, although a bit more specific, still happen in several places in the brain. For instance, endorphins are released by alcohol in the ventral tegmental area, the origin of the classic dopamine cells thought to make up a final common reward pathway. In that case the endorphin release triggered by alcohol is what activates the dopamine cells. But when alcohol is ingested, endorphins are also sent out at the brain site where this dopamine pathway ends, the nucleus accumbens, where they can activate that structure directly. There is also endorphin release in parts of the frontal lobes. These mechanisms, and then some, act together to let alcohol activate classical brain reward circuitry. The end results may be a bit counterintuitive. Despite being a brain depressant, alcohol can produce reward, positive reinforcement, and also a general stimulation of movement, or "psychomotor stimulation." But as already mentioned, it will ultimately also depress a wide range of brain processes.

These multifaceted effects of alcohol follow a two-phase progression. At the lower end of the intake spectrum, the rewarding and motor-stimulating effects tend to dominate, together with a dampening of anxiety that leads to behavioral disinhibition and a further accentuated, stimulant-like net result. The dampening effects begin to take over as higher amounts are consumed, leading to impairment, loss of balance, sleepiness, and ultimately unconsciousness. But because so many different actions combine to produce the net effect of alcohol on the brain, there is great potential for different people to be affected differently. Say, for instance, that for some reason, the cascade alcohol → endorphin → dopamine → reward and movement happens to be particularly responsive in your case. At the same time, perhaps your sensitivity to the dampening actions is low. In this scenario the rewarding and stimulant-like actions of alcohol will dominate up to very high intake levels.

For someone else maybe a mild reduction of tension and anxiety will directly be followed by becoming tired and sleepy. Genetics, sex, age, tolerance, and other "host factors" will in each case determine the relative contributions of the different alcohol effects to the net outcome. Perhaps most important, they will determine the balance between rewarding and motor-stimulating actions, on one hand, and dampening and sleep-inducing effects, on the other. As we will see when we come to medications for alcoholism, these distinctions are becoming increasingly important to understand.

And then, after exposing the brain for a long time to cycles of intoxication and withdrawal, the now familiar allostatic shift will occur. Alcohol may not be as intensely rewarding as other addictive drugs initially, but the allostatic process is probably more pronounced with this drug than with most if not all other addictive substances. In the presence of alcohol, opponent processes are progressively recruited that counteract acute alcohol actions. When alcohol is withdrawn, these opponent processes become predominant. For instance, processes opposing the dampening and sleep-inducing actions of alcohol, when uncovered, will result in the sometimes dramatic increase in nervous system excitability seen during alcohol withdrawal. This makes people jittery or anxious and can in more severe cases lead to withdrawal seizures and delirium tremens. Dialing up of processes that oppose the rewarding and motor-stimulating actions of alcohol actions will lead to a progressively dampened reward-system function: less dopamine, higher intracranial self-stimulation thresholds, all being signs of what can be called a reward deficit syndrome. Meanwhile, turned-up activity of corticotropin-releasing factor will further increase negative emotions and stress reactions. In the vicious circle characteristic of the dark side of addiction, this will set the scene for increased negative reinforcement through renewed alcohol intake.

15

TRICK OR TREATMENT

AM AT THE gym, staring at a television to break the monotony of the treadmill. A man, whose name I have since learned is Chris Prantiss, looks at me from the screen, slim and good-looking with his gray hair, suntan, and dark suit. He is standing next to his son, Pax, just as elegant himself. The older man has his hand affectionately placed on the younger man's shoulder. I hear him talk about the book he has written.

> I wrote *The Alcoholism and Addiction Cure* to give you hope and to share
> with you what works. Within the covers of my book, I will show you how
> to cure your addiction to alcohol, prescription drugs, street drugs, smok-
> ing, food addictions, sex addictions, gambling, and all other addictions.
> Notice that I do not say "however," "maybe," "although," "perhaps," or use
> other qualifying terms or conditions. By reading my book you will learn
> exactly how to cure your dependency. *The Alcoholism and Addiction Cure*
> contains the process that we use at the Passages Addiction Cure Center
> in Malibu, California. Passages currently has a very high success rate for
> curing all forms of addiction.[1]

Really. I guess I can close down my lab and start trying to figure out what to do. Which may be hard, because I really don't like to play golf.

Or maybe not. There are indeed a number of treatments for addictive disorders that have shown some degree of efficacy[2] in randomized controlled trials, the staple of evidence-based medicine. Famously invented by the Royal British Navy physician James Lind in the eighteenth century,[3] this is ultimately the only way to know if a treatment really does what it is claimed to do, in any field of medicine. It is therefore encouraging that the number of studies evaluating the efficacy of addiction treatments with this stringent methodology has steadily risen over the past three decades; all the while their scientific quality has also improved. A vast majority of this research in the world, probably more than 90 percent, is funded by American taxpayers, through the National Institutes of Health (NIH).[4] Based on this science, there is support for efficacy of both behavioral and pharmacological treatments.

It is also important at this stage to point out that treatment studies face many challenges. Even when carried out with the best possible methodology, there is ultimately a certain element of chance, which can skew the results of any single trial, one way or the other. That is why multiple studies at different sites are needed to properly evaluate a treatment. It is only once evidence from these multiple studies accumulates that one can start to feel really confident about having a reliable assessment of a treatment. Another staple of evidence-based medicine, the meta-analysis, is the technique for boiling down the results from these multiple studies to a unified picture. By that sophisticated approach, several behavioral treatments as well as addiction medications—methadone and buprenorphine for opioid addiction, the nicotine patch and varenicline for smoking cessation, naltrexone and acamprosate for alcoholism—are clearly effective.

Just *how* effective these treatments are is a separate issue. The conclusion that a treatment has a statistically significant effect means only that the difference in outcomes between treated patients and some appropriate comparison group is unlikely to have been caused by chance. It does not say anything about the magnitude of the clinical benefit produced. A treatment that has "significant" effects could therefore still be providing only a small, perhaps not really meaningful amount of improvement on average. An intuitively informative measure to express the amount of benefit is the "number needed to treat," or NNT:[5] how many patients will I need to treat, on average, to prevent an adverse outcome in a single individual? Methadone maintenance for preventing relapse to heroin addiction has one of the best NNTs in clinical medicine, below 2 in many of the better studies. For the most part, the effect sizes of other addiction treatments are modest but not necessarily all that inferior to widely accepted treatments in other areas of medicine. For instance, the NNT for the medication naltrexone to prevent relapse to heavy drinking is around 7, compared with an NNT of 3 for a widely prescribed beta-blocker to prevent exercise-induced chest pain, a treatment considered to be a major success story. On balance it would then seem that what we have is useful, while at the same time it is clear that we would like to do much better. The latter is of course what current research, including my own, tries to achieve.

Meanwhile, however, you would think there would be widespread use of the tools already available to us. After all, if a chemotherapy for some cancer form modestly improved five-year survival, say, from 12 to 25 percent, surely you would not shrug it off and do nothing, while waiting for the miracle drug that will save 90 percent of the patients?

And here is something else you would certainly not do, at least not in the case of cancer: you would not, instead, have patients sit in a circle and talk, drink carrot juice, take cleansing baths, be subject to herbal treatments, or receive other interventions based on nothing but a claim that in your experience, you have found these things to be helpful. Or at least you would not do this if you were a licensed physician, because if you did, the state medical board would quickly make sure that you would not remain one for long.[6] Yet the equivalent of exactly these things is going on day after day when it comes to the treatment of addictive disorders.

I started having my eyes opened to the discrepancy between what we should be offering patients and what is actually being done more than two decades ago, and I still recall the feeling of shock and disbelief. In 1989 Ried Hester and Bill Miller, legendary behavioral researchers at the University of New Mexico, published a book, the *Handbook of Alcoholism Treatment Approaches*, that attempted to bring together all the available evidence on the efficacy of alcoholism therapies and combined this with some deeply disturbing real-world observations.[7] The book was very useful as a whole, with the later chapters providing concise descriptions of important behavioral treatment approaches. But the first two chapters were what converted me from the all too common practice of "opinion-based medicine" to trying to make treatment choices informed by data. The book has subsequently been updated twice, the latest in 2003, but little has changed between the editions or since then.

What was so disturbing about this reading that it brought me out of my intellectual slumber? Three things stand out: First, as I have already said, there are treatments that do a modest but significant and useful amount of good in addictive disorders. As you will see, these treatments interact with the addiction mechanisms we have already covered. Conversely, there are treatments that have been evaluated by the same stringent methods and have consistently been shown to be ineffective. Second, in the analysis there was a significant *inverse* correlation between how well supported the efficacy of a treatment was and how much it cost. Overall the effective treatments were cheap, and the expensive ones were ineffective. This was rather provocative. The third observation was, however, the most disturbing. The treatments with documented efficacy and low cost were rarely provided to patients. The treatments with documented lack of efficacy and high cost were the ones most commonly offered.

I read and reread those chapters and vowed to rethink my ways. It was tough going because it forced me to reevaluate much that I thought I already knew and to learn many new things. I promised myself in those days that I would always come to work ready to change the way I practiced medicine if solid data suggested that was called for. One might think that would be a given in any field of medicine, but along the way I discovered that these insights were frequently met with indifference at best, and on many occasions with outright hostility. A few years later I became the director of a large addiction medicine service and was confronted with both the opportunity and the challenge of delivering care to large numbers of real patients who needed it. Together with a dedicated leadership team, we decided to revamp the whole service based on the available evidence. I had expected a lot of resistance from treatment staff, and there was certainly some of that. Less than a year into that work, however, most nurses and other treatment providers had in fact been bitten by the evidence bug and were helping drive the change themselves, curious about the best way to help patients they truly cared about. To my surprise and dismay, the hardest part instead turned out to be dealing with policy makers who just "knew" how addiction was to be treated, no matter what the data said. After all, we all have a cousin who drinks too much, don't we?

But neither when I was busy managing the treatment service nor when I ultimately retreated into a more academic existence did I pay enough attention to the megabuck industry that is based on provision of "treatment" that costs much and achieves little. These are businesses that promise a "cure" and charge astronomical amounts of money in ways that simply prey on people made vulnerable by their addictions. The industry obviously has a disincentive to provide inexpensive treatments that work. After all, these may ultimately prevent patients from coming back, and put the industry out of business.

Like most people who realize they have been taken for a ride, I was upset not only because of what was going on but also because I felt like a fool. Once I had a chance to think about it for a while, I decided to convert the energy of my frustration into something that could hopefully be more useful. So many lives are devastated by addictive disorders. So many of my colleagues work passionately to better understand and treat these conditions. Yet despite the advances this hard work has brought, very little has changed in the practice of addiction medicine outside academic settings. I am convinced that in order to bring much-needed change, patients, their loved ones, policy makers, and the public need to share the scientific advances the field has made. The individual news story that highlights an occasional new research finding may be great. But even when it is, it rarely provides the greater context in which every scientific advance happens or avoids the oversimplifications required by a short format. And too often the message becomes one of the sensation *du jour*—finding yet another "addiction gene," "addiction transmitter," or "cure." These stories rarely if ever fundamentally alter the way people view or handle the problems of addiction.

We need to do better. Only a better-informed public will become a more tolerant and caring public. Only better-informed patients will become less vulnerable patients.

In developed countries we tend to take advances of modern medicine for granted. It is easy to forget that until fairly recently the history of treating medical conditions isn't all that glorious. I don't know when exactly the scales tipped in favor of doing good over causing harm, but it is definitely less than a hundred years ago. Trepanation, the time-tested practice of drilling a hole in the skull as a treatment for brain disorders, continued to the Middle Ages, as documented in the famous Hieronymus Bosch painting *Extracting the Stone of Madness*. And bloodletting remained in practice as a treatment for fevers and infections throughout the nineteenth century. It most likely claimed the life of George Washington, who might have been able to deal with the throat infection he contracted in 1799 but definitively got in trouble after he was bled almost 4 liters.

With the benefit of hindsight, it is easy to find these methods absurd. My point is that, absent an understanding of disease mechanisms or data from randomized controlled trials, many approaches that at the time seem to make sense later turn out not to be very helpful. If you don't understand that social stress is a major relapse trigger in addiction, it may seem like a good idea to stage dramatic surprise confrontations between patients with addictive disorders and people affected by their behavior. If you fail to appreciate that patients with addictions apply steep temporal discounting to outcomes that are distant in time compared to those that are immediate, then you may want to spend a lot of time and money on educational movies that extol the dangers of alcohol use to the liver. I could go on, but you get the idea. And, by the way, in controlled trials, both the methods I just mentioned are of course entirely ineffective, as are standard addiction counseling, psychodynamic psychotherapy, and a host of other approaches that continue to be widely practiced, sometimes at great cost. In contrast, a number of behavioral as well as pharmacological methods that do produce measurable improvements still have not been implemented to the extent the data justify. A common theme is that these treatments all make sense in the context of the addiction mechanisms we have begun to uncover.

Of course, treatments need to be tailored to those being treated. A socially anxious, alcohol-dependent man who is medically healthy, is employed, and lives together with a loving family in a house in the suburbs will require different ingredients in his "treatment soup" than an impulsive, homeless heroin addict who has to steal for a living, has advanced hepatitis C, and is losing teeth. This is not a textbook to actually teach addiction treatment, but extensive research shows that we can't effectively treat patients with addictive disorders without carefully assessing their needs in the many areas of life where those needs exist. To properly tailor treatment, we need to take in account not only the nature and severity of the addictive disorder but also psychiatric and medical problems, housing, occupation, and crime, to mention those that are most important. This can clearly be done in many different ways, but research shows that systematic, structured approaches are the ones that work best. In their absence, even experienced treatment providers frequently find that they have failed to cover important areas of assessment. Believe me—been there, done that. More than three decades ago Tom McLellan, whom we met earlier in this book, developed the Addiction Severity Index (ASI).[8] This is an interview that typically takes less than an hour and covers what is important. The materials are free and have been translated into some thirty languages. I frankly cannot imagine running a treatment program without it.

A systematic assessment like the ASI or something along the same lines identifies areas in need of services and helps direct treatment efforts to those areas. But it does more than that. It serves a purpose just as important as any of the hardnosed science in this book. That purpose is to build a relationship with the patient, viewed as a fellow human being. That relationship in turn allows an alliance to be established. To paraphrase Kirkegaard, you can rarely help people arrive at a new place in life unless, for a while at least, you walk beside them. There is a terrible tradition of talking about addicts who relapse as showing "resistance to treatment," or not showing "motivation" for change. In fact, research shows that motivation is more a function of the interaction between the treatment provider and the patient. Walk into an office and say, "I have a solution for your problems, and it requires you to change," and you will experience resistance. Walk into the same office and ask, "What pains you?" and you will share an inner world and begin building a relationship with a person. Then the progression to asking more and more specifics will feel like—and be—a reflection of this intricate relationship web being woven. Once that is done, the work toward change can start, as a joint effort.

So we could say, "You are powerless under your addiction, and you should never again touch alcohol." Or, instead, we could listen for a while and then say, "You told me that even when you plan to take just one or two drinks, your drinking often spirals out of control. You told me that when that happens, you do things to your kids that make you feel terrible afterward. You know, many people I've worked with have told me that in the end, they found it easier to just avoid alcohol, rather than trying to control the amount they drink. Is that something you would consider trying for a while?" Although we are in both cases trying to work toward the same goal, research shows that the former approach will often meet resistance and lack of motivation. In contrast, the latter method will help the patient evolve toward a greater readiness for change, perhaps through intermediary goals that we can set up together, work toward, and evaluate. While all that happens, we are building something that is central to all treatment that requires behavioral change. To get to their goals, people need to feel that they have an ability to influence the course of their lives. Patients with addictions are no different. The feeling of this ability is the essence of the Stanford psychologist Albert Bandura's concept of "self-efficacy."[9] People who develop addictions frequently don't have much of that feeling to begin with. Addiction effectively degrades it further. Tragically, confrontational or coercive addiction treatments then add insult to injury.

This is the place where science and humanism come together in this book. There is a widespread perception that people who take an interest in neurotransmitters and their receptors, or who offer to treat ailments of the mind with medications, are cold cynics who don't care about their patient's feelings and "objectify" patients into some kind of guinea pigs. The clinical and human realities are instead that the two perspectives of science and humanism are inseparable in any area of medicine, but perhaps most so in psychiatry and addiction medicine. In a good addiction treatment program, humanism and science aid each other, as do empathy and anticraving medications. As I stated in a prior chapter, I don't know how to theoretically reconcile an understanding of the brain as a machinery that produces behavior based on the laws of nature, on one hand, with a view of the brain's owner as an agent endowed with a free will to choose one behavior over another, on the other. It does not seem that anyone else knows the answer to this dilemma either, so I have decided not to worry too much about it for now. But I do know this: patients with addictions strive toward and long for the same things that the rest of us do—love, work, a reasonable amount of material goods. And none of them wants to get sick or die from drugs. Those who say they do, as sometimes does happen, are really only saying, "To be alive like this is too painful." The problem addicts have is not that they strive toward taking drugs and all the bad things that leads to. The problem is that brain machinery that allows the rest of us to guide behavior toward better goals somehow is broken or overpowered in people with addictions, so that they end up taking drugs instead of achieving what they dream of.

I am saying all this to explain that any effective treatment has to reflect a marriage of two perspectives. One is more of a general framework than a specific method, although it is not without its own techniques. This is the perspective that is focused on building a relationship that allows the treatment provider to walk beside the patient. This perspective boils down to caring about and respecting the fellow human who also happens to be a patient. Clearly this is the domain of words spoken, but even more, of words listened to. The other perspective is about the specific, scientifically based methods for helping guide the course of this walk in a desired direction and actually getting there. That is the domain of science that provides specific tools and techniques to put at the disposal of our patients. Among useful tools, there are both those that are behavioral and those that are pharmacological. But in the end, it all has to come together. After all, what matters is behavior, and helping patients gain control over it so that it can take them where they want to be. And all that behavior is produced by brains.

16

PLEASE BEHAVE

OR ME, A general framework called motivational interviewing is a good bridge between the dialogue with the patient and the specific methods aimed at behavioral change. Motivational interviewing is, in its simplest form, a basic technique that should be used by anyone working with patients who have addictive disorders. Motivational enhancement therapy is an application of this technique toward specific treatment goals. Beneficial effects from these approaches are well supported by research.[1] In either shape, they are almost an antithesis to various confrontational methods. They bring together empathy and relationship-building principles that will be familiar to anyone with old-fashioned psychotherapy training, on one hand, and modern cognitive-behavioral strategies for achieving behavioral change, on the other.

Motivational interviewing and motivational enhancement therapy are based on the same principles. The first of these is expressing empathy. This may seem trivial, but here it takes on the specific form of reflective listening, expressing acceptance, and viewing the patient's ambivalence or reluctance to change as something normal. The second principle is to help develop discrepancy. "You told me you are all stressed out about being able to pay the electricity bills this month. But you also said that you spend a lot of money in the bar every weekend. Can we talk about that?" The third principle is to roll with what appears to be resistance rather than pushing against it and building it up even stronger. Finally, everything that is done in treatment is done to support the patient's self-efficacy. In the end, in order to succeed, people with addictions must take control of their own lives, just like a diabetic or any other patient with a chronic, relapsing disorder. In the long run, no patient can have a treatment provider help him or her make the thousands of decisions, big and small, that everyday life consists of. Avoiding immediate dangers, such as an overdose or suicide, can occasionally be coerced; long-term success cannot. Any treatment program that does not build on this insight diminishes people and is also less likely to be successful in the long run. People have to be in charge of their lives to change them. As one would expect, the feeling of self-efficacy is a good predictor of treatment outcomes.

I am not aware of any good research on the neural substrates of self-efficacy, but there is an attractive and testable hypothesis that articulates what the phenomenon probably is about at the level of brain circuits. As we have learned, frontocortical brain circuitry integrates the value of future outcomes with the need to adjust behavior, switch between different behavioral strategies, and suppress immediate impulses in order to achieve more highly valued outcomes that lie further into the future. It is not far-fetched to hypothesize that self-efficacy is a reflection of the efficiency with which the frontocortical circuitry does this job, in the process overriding impulsive, immediate reward- or relief-seeking behaviors. An extension of this hypothesis is that methods aimed at strengthening self-efficacy are based on approaching and practicing the same brain functions in ways that allow people to get better at them.

That is all good and well as a start. But as most of us know, even with the best of motivations, behavioral change is hard. Motivational interviewing and strengthening self-efficacy are a general framework, and a starting point to set the scene for change. More specific tools are needed to address behaviors that prevent people from changing drug-seeking behaviors. I will discuss those tools shortly. For starters, however, let's get something out of the way. Among specific intervention techniques to reduce harm from alcohol use in particular, some of the best data in the field are on a technique called brief intervention. This is as simple as it sounds. It could essentially consist of a physician seeing a patient, screening for alcohol use with a simple questionnaire such as the Alcohol Use Disorder Identification Test (AUDIT)[2] developed by the World Health Organization or a liver test, and having a single feedback session with the patient if there are indications of hazardous levels of consumption. Doing this in the context of a general practice has solid beneficial effects, both for drinking and for hard health-related outcomes, such as sick days or hospital admissions. Impressively, these effects may persist for several years. Research also shows that a single session is fine, and longer series of treatment sessions don't necessarily add up to better effects, although to maintain benefits, there seems to be a need for booster doses after some years.

The caveat with brief interventions is that policy makers and insurance companies often see them as a panacea for people with substance use problems, for obvious reasons. Brief interventions do not require a lot of resources compared to specialized addiction treatments and continuing recovery management that may have to last for years. Now, outcomes are all that matters, and there is no inherent value to seeing people in treatment month after month or year after year. But the caveat is that studies in which brief interventions show significant effects are typically carried out in general practice, where people have not specifically sought treatment for an addictive disorder. And the effect sizes observed in controlled studies on brief interventions are on average small to medium in people consuming alcohol. More important, they increase quite a bit if individuals with more severe alcohol problems are excluded. That tells us that brief interventions work primarily in people who may be high consumers and therefore benefit from cutting down but don't necessarily have an addictive disorder.[3] So, to sum up, this approach has tremendous potential to positively affect public health if broadly implemented in the general health care system. It is highly cost effective. I am all for it. Let's just not confuse it with addiction treatment.

How, then, can we bring together what we have learned about addiction—for instance, about mechanisms of reward, negatively reinforced drug use, impaired decision making, and relapse triggers—with effective treatment interventions? Describing in-depth specific, evidence-based approaches to treating addiction would obviously take up a whole book of its own. But all effective treatments have some key elements in common.[4] First, they all specifically focus on drug seeking and taking. Once again, this may sound trivial, but think back to the days of Edward Khantzian and self-medication views of addiction. Implicit in that view, still applied by many clinicians, was that if, for instance, underlying depression drives a person's alcoholism, then treating that depression will cure the alcoholism as well. It doesn't. Studies show that treating depression in people with alcoholism or drug addiction does lead to improvement of the depression symptoms but does not improve drinking outcomes.[5] Second, methods that focus on practicing changing specific behaviors do a better job than methods that talk about these behaviors, try to dissect intrapsychic conflicts thought to underlie them, or apply other complicated psychological constructs. Over my years as a clinician in behavioral health, I have learned a principle that applies quite broadly. If you want to help patients change the way they talk, help them talk. If you want to help them change the way they behave, help them carry out the behaviors. The modern version of William James's theory of emotions is "move your body, and your mind will follow." Third, all evidence-based addiction treatments intervene in the disease process in ways that make sense in the context of what we have so far learned about brain mechanisms of addiction and by doing so reduce the risk of relapse.

By now the chronic, relapsing nature of addictive disorders should be familiar, and so it should come as no surprise that preventing relapse is the central objective for addiction treatments that improve outcomes in measurable ways. This shines a bright light on an elephant in the room. There is an anomaly in the treatment of addictive disorders that simply will have to be fixed before we can do better than today. To the extent that addiction treatment is at all supported in the community, most of the resources continue to be devoted to "detoxification"[6] and other ways of initiating abstinence. Yet research uniformly shows that these interventions do not have a measurable impact on long-term outcomes in addictive disorders.

At one time it perhaps made more sense to devote a lot of attention to initiating abstinence, because this could be anything but trivial. A hundred years ago, suddenly discontinuing heavy alcohol use carried with it a considerable risk for precipitating a delirium tremens, a condition characterized by severe hyperexcitability of the entire nervous system. Most people have forgotten this now, but the tremors, hallucinations, and disorganized behaviors of this syndrome, accompanied by a risk for seizures, once carried with them a risk of dying that was about 20 percent. Getting off opioids, although in fact less dangerous, could nevertheless be an excruciating experience, a combination of a severe flu-like syndrome and fluids escaping from all glands of the body until, occasionally, severe dehydration would result. By now, however, we have long had ways of successfully and safely initiating abstinence from alcohol, opiates, and other drugs. Proper use of medication tapers, combined with some simple principles of supportive care, render this part of treatment almost trivial if properly managed.

The techniques to successfully manage withdrawal and initiate abstinence are of course major advances of addiction medicine. If a person dies from delirium tremens, then there is not much point in thinking much about long-term recovery. But despite our ability to safely initiate abstinence, somewhere around two-thirds of patients continue to relapse to drug use over the course of a year after detoxification, whether we look at alcohol, opioids, cocaine, or other drugs.[7] When they do, there is disappointment, frequently to the point that people—treatment providers, family members, patients themselves—give up. In fact, spending vast resources on repeatedly initiating abstinence and managing its early stages is most of the time a waste. What patients with addictive disorders need is chronic, perhaps life-long recovery management. And at the core of this long term disease management approach, they need methods that can help prevent relapse.

In fact, unless followed by effective long-term treatments, detoxifying people may make things worse. For instance, as mentioned in an earlier chapter, heroin addicts build up a high degree of tolerance while actively using drugs. To continue getting the desired drug effects, they progressively increase their heroin doses. When hospitalized or incarcerated and detoxified, they lose this tolerance within about a week. Yet when discharged after detoxification, patients, and in particular those among them who are young and not all that experienced, frequently return to the heroin doses they were using previously. Data from opioid addicts recently released from prison support what many of us have feared and suspected for a long time. When released after having lost their tolerance, these people run a much higher risk of dying from an overdose—sometimes as much as an eightfold increase—compared to people who just continued to use drug.[8] Although less well studied, it seems that multiple cycles of detoxification from alcohol can also be deleterious. They seem to push along the brain changes that are part of the addictive process and so contribute to the increasing motivation for drug seeking and taking.

So safely and humanely detoxifying people and initiating abstinence makes sense if it is a component in a well thought through, long-term plan for managing their addiction. Detoxifying patients and then thinking what to do next, if anything, puts the cart before the horse. Right there, I believe we saved at least half the money needed to fund evidence-based addiction treatment for a majority of people who now cannot afford it.

Specific behavioral methods to reduce relapse risk in addiction come in many flavors, but it is probably appropriate to highlight the contributions of Alan Marlatt, who spent most of his career at the University of Washington until he passed away in 2011.[9] Many others have of course contributed as well. Each variant of these techniques may have its own proponents who swear by it. To a large extent, however, these tools are, at least in principle, variations on the same themes taken from the playbook of cognitive behavioral therapy and applied to the various phenomena of addiction already discussed in this book.[10] It will not take me long to explain the basics of behavioral relapse prevention treatments.

First and foremost, however, in an established tradition of behavioral therapy, we have to work with patients to break down the process that leads up to relapse into its behavioral elements. Frequently the patient perceives relapse as a black box, an incomprehensible disaster, or a lightning bolt out of a blue sky. When I go into an exam room, I frequently hear something along these lines: "Here I was, almost six months sober, thinking things were mostly back on track. And then this. It is terrible. I've lost it all. Don't know what got into me. I am powerless. Might just as well give up." Not a lot of self-efficacy there. A while later, however, the story often turns out to be rather different. "Things were pretty much fine. Then we got this big new order at work. No one wanted to say it, but we really didn't have the capacity to take it on. After a while, the whole office got behind. As the deadline approached, there was more and more infighting, blaming, and finger pointing. One day somehow everyone ended up beating up on me. I didn't take it too seriously at first, but then, on the way home, little things I normally don't worry about started bothering me. When I just missed a connection, I thought I was going to scream. Once I caught the next one and finally got to my stop, I somehow decided to walk home from the metro instead of taking the shuttle bus. There is this bar along the way that I had totally forgotten about. I was really surprised to find myself outside of it. Then I thought, I'll just go in and sit here for while and find some composure before I go home, or my wife will start to worry that something is wrong. I remember, after the first three drinks, I realized this is going to hell. Then I thought, it is pointless to try. I never came home that night."

What may appear to the patient as an incomprehensible black hole is in fact a progression of small, logical steps. Many times when cravings are triggered, for instance, when they are set off by social stressors, the patient does not consciously realize it. A fight within the family or at work is among the most common ways it happens, but there is often an interesting delay before this leads to cravings, making the connection less obvious. Once the cravings are triggered, they generate a subtle attentional bias to drug-related memories and cues. In small steps, this bias guides behavior in directions where sooner or later there will be an opportunity to resume drug taking. Once that happens, the powerful reinforcing properties of the drug take over, be they rewarding, relieving, or, most of the time, both. In the absence of well-practiced behavioral strategies, the sophisticated but fragile frontocortical machinery that handles valuation of outcomes, decision making, and task switching now becomes overpowered. And once that happens, there is a particular kind of catastrophic thinking. "All is lost. There is no point in even trying."

The steps below are ones I advise patients to follow to deal with relapse.

1. Identify your own relapse triggers. These tend to have common themes, but in the lives of real people, they always come with a personal flavor. If

you are a socially anxious person, then the kind of antagonistic social inter-action I just described tends to set you off. But even within that category, there is much variety. Our bonds with children, spouses, or colleagues can all be tremendously important social rewards. For that very reason, they are also potential sources of a terrible social threat, when the strings of attach-ment look like they are at risk of being damaged or severed. But not all relapse triggers are related to negative emotionality. Other people may be more sensitive to positive feeling as relapse triggers. In talking about this, a fascinating paper by my colleagues Kenzie Preston and David Epstein at the National Institute on Drug Abuse always comes to mind. To track people with addictions in the real world of Baltimore, they let their subjects use handheld electronic devices and had them continuously register what was going on. The idea was that if the subjects relapsed, it would be possible to analyze what events had preceded their drug taking. For relapse to heroin use, stress and negative emotionality indeed turned out to be the most com-mon antecedents of relapse. But for cocaine, the research team identified a different pattern, one for which they coined the equally innovative and tell-ing term "celebratory relapse."[11]

2. Once you've written the list of things that are your personal relapse triggers and written down the chains of small steps that lead from those triggers to drug taking, start developing a set of screenplays for the movie of your own life, screenplays that have another kind of ending. The famous Shakespeare line "All the world's a stage, and all the men and women merely players" may be true, but you can also be the screenwriter and the director. For starters, develop a script, or in fact a number of them, that avoid the situations triggering cravings and relapse. Use your creativity to develop what that alternative plot will be, because it has to be one that works for you, and you are the expert on your own life. But the important thing is that once you have developed those scripts, you'll have to do what any actor who wants to get really good must do: practice. And practice. And practice again. Remember, not talk about it, but rather do it. And because most of the scripts will be of interactions with other people, you will have to practice together with others. Hence relapse prevention lends itself unusually well to a group format. Group members can put each other to great use by practicing

behavioral strategies in the form of role-playing. Incidentally, the group format also renders treatment highly cost effective.

3. You will not always succeed in avoiding relapse triggers. Life is, after all, not predictable to a degree that would allow you to prepare a script for every situation you may encounter. And even in familiar situations, your performance may not always be perfect. For that reason you will also have to prepare strategies for situations when cravings do get triggered. Of course, along the way, you will have to learn how to recognize them. By the time you actually think, "I need a drink," it is probably quite late. In talking to spouses of alcoholics and drug addicts, I have been amazed how well they can see the early signs that cravings are on the rise even though the patient still does not seem to have an idea what is going on. There is perhaps some aimless wandering, and a certain degree of irritability. There may be a desire for sweets or other foods. There may be something else that is unique to you. Once you have learned to recognize those signs, learn how to pay attention to them. Bring them into your conscious thoughts and hold them there. Be mindful of them. And then learn to cope with them. One of the best coping strategies is learning to do nothing for a while. The secret is that craving, just as anxiety, dissipates over time. Patients with anxiety disorders discover that, if they can avoid being engulfed in panic and run away, their distress tapers off. This is an extremely powerful experience. It can initiate new learning that over time results in extinction of the fears. Craving is very similar in this respect. In fact, extinction of fear and cravings seems to be driven by brain circuitry that is closely interconnected.[12] As a standalone treatment, cue exposure and coping skills therapy, pioneered by Peter Monti at Brown University, is an example of this of approach. It uses techniques that actively elicit cravings to help patients learn the skills to successfully cope with them.[13]

4. It is never too late. Just because you did not stop after the first drink does not mean you have less reason to stop after the second, or third. And even a full-blown relapse is not the end of the world. Hopefully, if you have applied the techniques outlined above, it took longer from the last relapse to this one than it took between the previous two. That is actually a good sign. Now, let's see how you can do better still. As unfortunate as a relapse

is, it is only to be expected in a chronic, relapsing disorder. So anyone view-ing it as a failure that invalidates prior treatment efforts is simply showing that they do not get what addiction is about. Once people—patients, family member, employers, those in the legal system—get past that level of igno-rance, we will all be in a better place. Rather than ruminating over relapse as a disaster, we will be able to see what lessons can be learned from it each time. What was the chain of behavioral steps that led up to it? What are the screenplays—the behavioral strategies—that need to be written to come to a different ending next time? How can those be practiced?

5. Remember the principles of reinforcement. If drug effects are pretty much the only reinforcers available to you, no one, and you yourself least of all, should be shocked that sooner or later you will use drugs. So we need to work on finding other reinforcers that can compete. Once again, this can be a component of an integrated behavioral relapse prevention approach, or it can be developed into standalone treatments. In the latter format, sev-eral approaches have been established and evaluated, with some of the best results in treatment of addictive disorders.[14] In one of these approaches, called voucher-based reinforcement therapy, patients receive vouchers with different monetary value for demonstrating sobriety or being abstinent from drugs. To promote continuous abstinence, the value of these vouchers is increased the longer clean urines or breathalyzer tests are produced. In another technique, called fishbowl reinforcement, clean urines or breath-alyzer tests are reinforced by receiving draws, often from slips of paper kept in a fishbowl, for providing a negative biological specimen. Typically about half the draws just say "Good job!" The other half result in the earning of a prize, which may range in value from $1 to $100. Again, to promote con-tinuous abstinence, clients receive bonus draws after a certain number of consecutive negative samples. While reinforcers must have a value that can compete with the reinforcement from drugs, that value does not necessar-ily have to be monetary. For patients in methadone maintenance, receiving take-home medication for longer intervals instead of coming to the clinic to receive medication every day is valuable because it allows them to live a more normal life. Other adaptations of this approach use housing or even fun activities as reinforcers.

In the end, the truly valuable things in life are of course outside of the treatment setting altogether. What really has value is family, friends, and all the other healthy pleasures of life. When relapse episodes no longer disrupt life on a regular basis, it is therefore time to get to work on setting up the right contingencies for a real, rewarding life. It is then about writing the scripts in which staying away from drugs and alcohol leads to greater rewards from real people who play the important roles in the screenplay of your life. Unless that happens, coming out of the haze of more or less chronic intoxication will just result in emptiness and sadness over things destroyed and things missing, rather than satisfaction. Take my word for it, if that is the case, then it will not be long before drugs start playing a major role in your life once again.

Motivational interviewing, CBT-based relapse prevention, and contingency management are all useful, solid techniques. They have been around for a while, and you may ask what, if anything, may lie beyond them. A recent wave of psychological approaches broadly covered by the umbrella term of "mindfulness" or "third-wave cognitive behavioral therapies" has more recently entered the psychotherapeutic stage and may indeed offer some useful tools. We are here not talking literally about the mindfulness that in the teachings of Buddha is one of the seven tools to reach enlightenment. This is a much more secular and practical version. In the early 1980s the techniques Buddhist meditation uses to reach mindfulness and enlightenment were adapted for psychological treatment by Jon Kabat-Zinn of the University of Massachusetts Medical School. Applied to reduction of everyday stress among busy, fundamentally healthy people, these techniques have become quite the vogue. For at least two decades, there has also been an interest among cognitive behavioral therapists in exploring whether these tools might be useful in the treatment of psychiatric disorders as well.

A key element of mindfulness training that might come in particularly handy in the treatment of addiction is to increase awareness of one's own thinking. We have already seen how much of the mental processes that lead up to relapse happen almost automatically, outside of one's awareness. Clearly, techniques that practice the ability to "be in the moment" and heighten awareness of one's own thoughts could hold the promise of catching early stages of thought processes leading up to relapse and changing their direction. But as always when appealing concepts are held up as new cures, we need to be cautious and stick close to the data. It is one thing for me to find mediation helpful in dealing with the stresses of working for a government agency. It is something altogether different to provide evidence of treatment effects in addiction. In fact, the only area where some data on mindfulness-based treatments are beginning to emerge is depression. The first meta-analysis of controlled studies that applied these approaches to depression treatment came out in 2013.[15] The conclusion was that mindfulness-based treatments may be as good as regular cognitive-based therapy, but there was no evidence that they would be any better. The evidence available so far was also deemed to be limited in amount and of low quality. In the field of addiction, there is even less solid data.

So what is, in the big picture, the future of behavioral treatments for addiction? My personal view is that the bottle is half full, half empty, and likely to stay that way. What I mean is that we have come a long way. The proper use of the evidence-based behavioral techniques reviewed in this chapter is clearly of help for people with addictive disorders. But more and more evidence suggests that increasingly sophisticated and intensive behavioral approaches, while costly to deliver, are not getting us much further. Perhaps a reasonable conclusion is that we may have gotten as far as it is reasonable to hope by applying behavioral treatments. We need to make sure that these are provided to people who need them. But we also need to look beyond them.

17

PILLS FOR ADDICTION ILLS

WHEN I WAS still in medical school, one of my instructors asked me what I wanted to do after I finished my training. I answered that I wanted to develop better treatments for people with addiction. He said, "Oh, you want to be a psychotherapist? Do you really need medical school for that?" I said no, I had seen people attend therapy for years while continuing to take drugs, and ultimately succumbing to them. I wanted to understand the brain mechanisms gone awry in addiction and see if we could do better, by finding medications that could somehow help those mechanisms get back on track. The instructor just shook his head. "Young man, how can you ever hope to treat a chemical addiction with yet another chemical?" This conversation has stuck with me. In endless variations, the statement is one I have since encountered countless times.

The statement was, of course, demonstrably wrong already at the time. Only four years later, in 1988, Vincent Dole of Rockefeller University in New York received the Lasker Medical Research Award for a medication that came to save countless lives and continues to do so. Here is the citation from the Lasker jury:

> In 1964, Dr. Dole, a distinguished authority on human metabolism and the treatment of obesity, recognized heroin addiction as a growing public

health problem that could not be solved by law enforcement, moralistic arguments, or traditional psychiatry. Making a completely new professional commitment, he began studying the physiological nature of chemical dependency.

Using a synthetic, long-acting opiate known as methadone, he discovered that carefully titrated doses of methadone could block an addict's craving for heroin during withdrawal, and that long-term methadone treatment provided a way for the addict to escape from the devastating cycle of heroin addiction.

He postulated that methadone blocked the sites in the brain where heroin would ordinarily act. He reasoned that the normal brain must include these receptor sites for normal neurotransmitter molecules. Years before technology was devised to study these sites, now known as endorphin receptors,[1] Dr. Dole conceived a laboratory protocol for their detection, and mathematically determined the number of endorphin receptors present in the brain.

With his wife and colleague, the late Marie Nyswander, Dr. Dole proved that heroin addicts could be regarded as patients with a chronic metabolic condition. When addiction is treated medically, antisocial and criminal behavior can be eliminated, and lives and resources can be saved. Methadone maintenance alone restores half those treated to useful life; when social and psychological support are supplied, the rate of success increases significantly.

Although heroin addiction may seem like an extreme, methadone is a good place to start a discussion of medications for addictive disorders, for a couple of reasons. First, it provided the first proof-of-principle that an addiction could indeed be effectively treated with a medication. Second, and perhaps even more important, methadone maintenance illustrates the importance of the addiction mechanisms detailed earlier in this book and shows how those can be targeted with medications. The changes in brain function I earlier labeled allostatic neuroadaptations are lasting shifts in the baseline of the brain's reward and stress systems. Once these shifts are in place, patients are miserable in the absence of drugs. They crave drugs both to get rid of that negative emotional state and to reexperience the high. Drugs such as heroin mimic the actions of endogenous morphine-like substances, or the endorphins, and activate the mu-opioid receptors through which these act to produce pleasure and suppress pain. But because it is so short acting, heroin potently triggers allostatic neuroadaptations, by first bombarding the mu-opioid receptors with a high intensity, then quickly coming off them. In contrast, methadone is extremely long acting. When adequately dosed, it is able to slowly activate the opioid receptors to the point of normalizing the patient's state and suppressing craving for a long time. At the same time, it prevents the patient from experiencing the high from heroin should he or she still try it. Both effects work together to prevent relapse.

Methadone is probably the most prominent example I know where preconceived notions for a long time got in the way of seeing what was in the data. For many years, countless people died from heroin addiction when they could have been successfully treated, only because people chose opinion-based medicine over the evidence-based variety. From its beginnings at the Rockefeller and for years to come, the use of methadone was mired in controversy, outlawed, capped, or looked down on, often by people who claimed to have the interest of heroin addicts in mind. This is not the book to detail those controversies. Over the years, numerous scientists brought clarity to this field. Among those, two Dole trainees had a particularly prominent role. Mary Jeanne Kreek, who continues to run a highly productive addiction research center at the Rockefeller, provided much of the insights into the mechanisms of methadone action. For decades she was also an outspoken and remarkably effective advocate for treatment, in the United States and worldwide. Lars Gunne, a Swedish psychiatrist, once came to the Rockefeller to learn novel, advanced chemistry techniques but realized the breakthrough nature of the methadone discovery. After returning home, he become the chair of psychiatry in Uppsala and went on to generate some of the most compelling data on the efficacy of methadone maintenance, combining it with a comprehensive psychosocial treatment.

By now the data are indisputable. Methadone maintenance effectively helps people stay in treatment and reduce their heroin use.[2] It is consistently better than various control conditions, even when the methadone treatment is bare bones and has few other elements besides the medication. However, the outcomes vary markedly between programs and studies and become progressively better with increased intensity of psychosocial treatment.[3] As a rule of thumb, in the absence of methadone maintenance, no more than 10 percent of patients are still in treatment after six months to a year, no matter how slow the detox from heroin, or how intensive the psychosocial treatment offered.[4] When methadone is provided, even with little or no psychosocial treatment, retention in treatment is typically about 50 percent over the same time frame. In the best programs, those that combine methadone maintenance with intensive psychosocial treatment, the way Gunne's program has always done in Uppsala, the corresponding number can reach 75 percent or better.[5] Over the years, when data like these were presented internationally, they were often met with disbelief. Surely outcomes of treating heroin addiction, one of the most deadly addictions, just could not be that good. Maybe the results somehow reflected a selection of less severely addicted patients? Maybe there was something special about breathing the air in Uppsala?

I learned most of what I know about opioid maintenance treatment from Lars Gunne, one of the most generous, caring, and brilliant people I have ever met. Several years after we had first been in touch and he gently started to instill in me his wisdom, my group applied his treatment principles to a population of unselected heroin addicts, literally taken right off the street. As much as I admired and respected Lars, I was still amazed to see that we got results very similar to those he had obtained.[6] The differences between programs are important to properly understand differences in outcomes beyond simply staying in treatment or reducing heroin use. Staying in treatment is just an indirect marker of success. What we really want to achieve is, first and foremost, that people don't die. After that, we want to facilitate change so that patients don't remain trapped in crime and prostitution. When all different methadone studies are put together in a meta-analysis, a reduction in mortality and crime rates is seen only as a trend, one that does not reach statistical significance. However, in studies with the better outcomes, such as those from Gunne's program, both death and crime rates are robustly reduced.[7] Perhaps one way of saying this is that methadone alone provides an opportunity to stay off heroin. The addition of psychosocial treatment provides the opportunity to make use of that pause from heroin to change one's life.

Yet methadone maintenance is not without its challenges. On the physician's part, it takes a while to teach people how to safely start up and manage the treatment. There are also some side effects that, although typically mild, can be problematic in a treatment that frequently needs to last many years or even decades. Almost all methadone patients become constipated, and quite a few become drowsy, so much so at times that this gets in the way of rehabilitation. The most important issue by far, however, is the risk for accidental overdose and death. Patients in methadone treatment develop tolerance to the medication and end up receiving daily doses—typically 70 to 120 mg—that will easily kill a person without tolerance, by suppressing their breathing. The risk is particularly high if people inject the methadone solution. Because of the overdose risk, great effort has to be devoted in any methadone program to prevent diversion of medication to illicit street use. In the early stages of treatment, patients have to visit a methadone clinic daily to receive their dose because their lives have not yet stabilized to the point that they can take responsibility for bringing a potentially deadly drug with them outside the clinic. Even once patients have been stable for a long time, most programs would hesitate to send along medication for more than perhaps two weeks. After years of successful treatment, by which time most patients are back to work, this creates unwelcome restrictions. And resources devoted to preventing diversion would of course be better used to treat more people.

In the 1990s a unique partnership among government, academia, and industry[8] brought to market a treatment for heroin addiction that has many of the advantages of methadone maintenance while addressing several of its downsides. Buprenorphine was first developed, in the 1970s, as a somewhat unusual pain suppressant. Similar to methadone, it is long acting and activates mu-opioid receptors, but it does so with a twist. It is what pharmacologists call a partial agonist. This means that like any drug similar to morphine or endorphins, buprenorphine recognizes the mu-opioid receptors and binds to them. The difference is that once buprenorphine is sitting on the receptor, it only partially activates it. This partial activation is most of the time sufficient to eliminate or at least reduce cravings for heroin, but it is not strong enough to give the patient much of a high or to suppress breathing. It does not matter how much the patient takes. The way partial agonists work, beyond a certain level, irrespective of the dose, there will not be more of an effect. We have reached a plateau. This means that the medication is easy to manage, is very safe to use, and does not pose an overdose risk, at least not as long as it is not mixed with a lot of other drugs. As a bonus, buprenorphine becomes even more tightly bound to the mu-opioid receptor than methadone. This means that it is better at blocking a possible high from heroin.

Just like one would expect from all this, stringent clinical studies showed that buprenorphine was highly effective as a treatment for heroin addiction,[9] something that has since been confirmed by numerous controlled trials.[10] The high safety and ease with which buprenorphine can be managed may sound mostly like a technicality, of interest only for the prescribing physician. In fact, in the real world, it has translated into tremendous opportunities for expanding access to treatment. Just as an example, when my group introduced buprenorphine in Sweden, only about 10 percent of heroin addicts there were in methadone maintenance treatment, waitlists were long, and people died while waiting to be admitted into treatment. When buprenorphine was introduced, waitlists were quickly shortened or eliminated, many times without the addition of any new treatment resources. By now close to 40 percent of Swedish heroin addicts receive treatment, half of them with buprenorphine.[11] In the United States the Food and Drug Administration approved buprenorphine for opioid addiction treatment in 2002, and the development was very similar. For the first time, it was now possible for a physician to take a course and then provide maintenance treatment to patients in his or her office, rather than in a traditional methadone program. The ease and lower cost of delivering treatment under these conditions quickly translated into a major expansion of treatment. A study from Yale University also showed that, just as one would expect, office-based treatment was able to attract people who otherwise had found treatment in a traditional program too stigmatizing to seek it out.[12]

A particularly clever use of simple pharmacological principles further minimized the diversion risk associated with buprenorphine treatment. Buprenorphine is taken under the tongue, from where it is taken up into the bloodstream. This route of absorption is far too slow to result in a high. But if someone really wanted to use buprenorphine to get a high, they could still try to dissolve it and inject the solution. To prevent this, a formulation was created in which buprenorphine was mixed with the opioid antidote naloxone. If naloxone is taken by mouth, it gets broken down in the liver before it has a chance to reach the brain.[13] So as long as patients are using their buprenorphine-naloxone combination as they are supposed to, the naloxone ingredient simply doesn't make a difference. But if the medication is injected intravenously, then the liver is bypassed. Both naloxone and buprenorphine now reach the brain. Naloxone blocks the opioid receptors and prevents buprenorphine from causing any receptor activation. Thus this is a package that retains its ability to effectively treat an otherwise deadly addiction but now has a markedly reduced overdose risk compared to methadone.[14]

The development of buprenorphine is a major success story of government, academia, and a drug company working together. The clinical benefits have been tremendous. With that as a background, this is perhaps the time to stick out my neck and say one more thing. Over the years, I have carefully guarded my independence from any drug company interests. To be credible, particularly in a field as contentious as this one, one simply cannot at the same time have a vested financial interest in any drug company, and its successes.[15] But many people fail to appreciate that the realities of pharmaceutical research in the field of addiction are very different from those in other therapeutic areas, those that the industry considers profitable.

Marketing departments of pharmaceutical companies typically do not consider addiction medications to be worth pursuing. Because of that, the prevailing stigma, and concerns about risks involved in treating this complicated population, the problem we have in the addiction field is not too much pharma involvement—it is too little. With the exception of smoking cessation treatments, it continues to be very difficult to engage the pharmaceutical industry to develop medications for addictive disorders. That is a major barrier that results in very little translation of scientific advances in the addiction field into new treatments. Academia and government agencies can do many of the steps involved in medication development well. But there are other parts of this process that simply require the involvement of the pharmaceutical industry. In this context, it is important to point out that buprenorphine, in addition to saving countless lives, has also been a commercial success. Contrary to common perceptions, there is a market for effective, safe medications for addictive disorders. The partial agonism properties of buprenorphine are, by the way, probably attractive beyond the treatment of heroin addiction. We will revisit them when we get back to smoking cessation.

Before we move away from medications for heroin addiction, I still have to introduce a molecule that I will have reason to spend more time with when discussing alcoholism medications. Naltrexone is a chemical relative of naloxone, but as opposed to its cousin, it can be taken by mouth and still reach the brain. Just like naloxone, naltrexone is a blocker, or "antagonist," for opioid receptors. This means that, just like methadone or buprenorphine, it will bind tightly to opioid receptors but without activating them at all. Because the receptors are now occupied by an inactive molecule, patients can inject as much heroin as they wish. They will not experience a high no matter what. The receptor is blocked.

If experiencing the high were all there was to heroin addiction, a daily dose of naltrexone would be a great treatment for this condition. It is not. Because naltrexone does not result in any receptor activation, heroin-dependent patients continue to experience intense cravings, until most of them discontinue the medication and relapse to heroin use. Overall, outcomes with naltrexone for heroin addiction are no better than without treatment. As one would expect when compliance is the key issue for treatment success, the medication has shown some positive effects in studies where patients have been forced to follow naltrexone treatment, for example, as a provision of their parole.[16] To improve compliance in other patient populations, injectable depot formulations of naltrexone have also been tried, so that the patient "only has to make one good decision a month." Short-term results with those formulations have been encouraging.[17] These results have been obtained by some of the best people in the field, whose judgment I have tremendous respect for. These colleagues are convinced that depot nal-trexone is a treatment approach with a good potential in heroin addiction. I hope they are right. Yet knowing how difficult heroin cravings are to endure, I am skeptical whether patients will keep coming back year after year, unless they receive a treatment that dampens those cravings. And if they don't come back for the next injection, the risk of relapse is there again.

Finally, to put medications for opioid addiction in context, it is impor-tant to realize that the face of this condition has been changing over time. Once, this therapeutic area was dominated by the need to treat severe cases, typically intravenous heroin addicts, many of whom had been recruited into drug use in the 1970s. Methadone maintenance, despite its challenges and the need for years or a lifetime of treatment, was usually appropriate in those cases, and that remains to be the case. Then there was a wave of new recruit-ment into opioid use among young people. It was not clear whether a deci-sion to initiate methadone maintenance in an eighteen-year-old after a year or two of irregular heroin smoking could be justified. Yet at the same time, a failure to provide this treatment could mean that the patient would die of an overdose the next day. Buprenorphine offers an attractive treatment for this group. Finally, over the past decade, the United States has experienced a continuous rise in nonmedical use of prescription opioid analgesics. These medications act at the same brain receptors as heroin and are highly addic-tive. It is currently estimated that close to two million people in the United States meet abuse or dependence criteria for this substance class. Their use accounts for a larger number of overdose deaths than those from heroin and cocaine combined, or about twelve thousand each year.

With this changing panorama, I think that there is a need for a progres-sion of treatments that can be tailored to the different levels of problem severity. Buprenorphine and methadone offer a logical progression that can be systematically followed. Buprenorphine, the safer, more easily managed medication, can be offered first. Even if it is somewhat less effective, it is reasonable to always try it first, just like penicillin should first be tried for pneumonia before using a broad spectrum antibiotic. If the patient does well on buprenorphine as first-line treatment, as about half the patients do, then the challenges of providing methadone treatment can be avoided.

If, on the other hand, the first-line treatment is insufficient, then a rapid transfer to methadone can be offered. This approach maximizes the benefits while minimizing the risks and the downsides.[18] Ideally, however, we would also like to have an option for cases where even initiating buprenorphine might seem questionable. In those cases, a medication without an addiction liability of its own would be ideal. Depot naltrexone may to some extent fill that niche. But if my hunch is correct and many patients will not stick with that treatment, then we should work hard to find other options.

In this book I have so far largely stayed away from smoking, other forms of nicotine addiction, and their treatment. As I pointed out at the beginning, there is no question that these disorders cause a tremendous disease burden, one that in aggregate takes a not-so-proud first position on the list of addictions. I have also mentioned that I have a couple of excuses for avoiding these important conditions. First, they are in a way a special case, in that the addictive drug nicotine, as such, is not particularly harmful. The harm is caused when motivation to obtain nicotine serves as an incentive for consumption of harmful products such as cigarettes. That is clearly different from, say, heroin addiction. Second, nicotine, as opposed to other addictive drugs, does not cause an immediate mental impairment. It improves cognitive function and is happily accessed, for instance in the form of nicotine gum, by some of my most responsible colleagues when they write important papers. Third, tobacco products, although regulated and equipped with warnings, remain legal. Combined, these differences have resulted in smoking cessation traditionally being offered outside my world of addiction medicine. And so I have to confess that I don't have much hands-on experience from treating nicotine addiction. Having said that, it is rather clear that much of what applies to treatment of other addictions is also true of nicotine. This is certainly also true for pharmacological treatment, in ways that will nicely echo the principles just covered for treatment of heroin or other opioid addiction.

In brief, the principle of maintenance treatment to some extent works for smoking as well. The logic of that principle is to use a slow-onset and long-lasting stimulation of the same receptors that the addictive drug itself otherwise activates with rapid on-off dynamics. The brain receptor to target for smoking cessation is the nicotinic acetylcholine receptor, whose activation ultimately turns on classical dopaminergic brain-reward circuitry. Nicotine addicts certainly display an allostatic shift of their affective and hedonic balance after extensive drug use, leaving them miserable when abstinent. To have a vivid illustration of that state, one need only to talk to someone who is trying to quit. In this case, the nicotine patch provides the equivalent of a methadone effect, although the slow dynamics in this case are the result of the slow-release patch delivery replacing smoking. Of course it helps that nicotine as such is reasonably benign. A recent meta-analysis that included studies carried out in some forty thousand people found that the nicotine patch, or "nicotine replacement therapy," improves chances of quitting by 50–70 percent.[19] This seems to be the case irrespective of what behavioral treatments replacement therapy is combined with. Once again, maintenance with a medication that fully activates the target receptor works.

And so does "maintenance" with a partial nicotinic agonist, a principle similar to buprenorphine for opioid addiction. In 2006 the Food and Drug Administration approved the partial nicotinic receptor agonist varenicline, sold in the United States as Chantix and in the rest of the world, oddly enough, as Champix. It seems that varenicline is able to activate nicotinic receptors in the brain enough to suppress cravings for nicotine. However, in an analogy to buprenorphine, if the patient attempts to smoke, the receptors are already occupied by the medication. This makes smoking or other attempts to obtain nicotine effects largely meaningless. Just as one would expect from these properties, varenicline is a robustly effective smoking-cessation medication.[20] It is less clear why, in this case, the partial agonist is *more* effective than maintenance with the fully active agonist nicotine itself. One possibility is that the cravings for nicotine, pronounced though they may be, perhaps are not as intense as cravings for opioids, making the receptor blockade relatively more important for treatment success.

Finally, you may wonder if there is a smoker's equivalent to naltrexone, which would block nicotinic receptors in nicotine addicts. Indeed there is. Mecamylamine is the right kind of nicotinic antagonist and has been tested for its ability to improve quit rates in smokers.[21] It actually did help. Having read about how hard it is to make opioid addicts stick with their antagonist treatment, you will perhaps not be entirely surprised to learn that no pharmaceutical company has so far pursued developing this or any other antagonist, despite the gigantic market for smoking cessation.

Medications for treatment of alcoholism unfortunately do not follow the appealing logic of opioid or nicotine addiction treatments. That was perhaps only to be expected. After all, opioids and nicotine target highly specific neurotransmitter systems, in each case with an established role in the motivational circuitry of the brain. In contrast, alcohol does not directly interact with any specific brain receptor. It was long thought to affect the brain in entirely nonspecific ways, by acting as a detergent of sorts on fat layers from which membranes of all cells are made. It turns out that is not how it works. As I have described, alcohol influences several major neurotransmitter systems of the brain, including opioids, dopamine, glutamate, and GABA.[22] It is hard to know which of those effects that should be targeted for treatment. To make matters worse, as mentioned previously, people differ in their responses to alcohol, based, among other things, on family history. This probably reflects genetic differences in how much different neurotransmitter systems contribute to a person's alcohol response. The contributions probably also vary depending on the person's sex, age, or stage of addiction. No wonder it has been difficult to develop effective medications for "alcoholism." If we consider these individual differences, developing medications that are helpful for every patient may simply not be a reasonable expectation. I am convinced that, as new medications get developed, one of the most important tasks will be to identify the optimal intervention for every patient from a menu of possible options.[23]

Before discussing neuropharmacological treatments for alcoholism, I need to briefly mention the alcoholism medication that is probably still best known to the public. Disulfiram, discovered in the 1920s, continues to be marketed, under the trade name Antabuse. Disulfiram does not intervene in the motivational mechanisms underlying alcoholism at all. Instead it simply blocks a step along the sequence through which alcohol is broken down and eliminated from the body. As a result of this blockade, the toxic substance acetaldehyde accumulates in the bloodstream. This in turn results in an extreme version of the Asian flush syndrome discussed in the genetics chapter. What that means is that if alcohol is consumed while a patient is on disulfiram, the accumulation of acetaldehyde results in facial flushing, as well as an extremely unpleasant and potentially dangerous reaction that includes a pounding heart and elevated blood pressure. This is intended to deter alcohol use, but of course it does nothing to reduce cravings for alcohol. If those cravings become too difficult to manage, the patient is still able to discontinue the medication and to relapse. As one would expect from this, disulfiram, offered as a prescription without supervised administration, is no more effective as a treatment than is placebo. It does, however, have some degree of efficacy if the medication is given in a supervised fashion, with a nurse watching and making sure that the patient actually takes the tablets every day.[24]

The first medication approved for the treatment of alcohol addiction that can be considered modern, in that it acts on the brain, is one discussed in the opioid treatment chapter, naltrexone. In 1980 it was reported that when naltrexone was given to eight rhesus monkeys, it suppressed their alcohol drinking at doses that did not significantly affect water consumption.[25] Influenced by these data, Chuck O'Brien and his colleagues at the Philadelphia VA Medical Center in 1983 obtained approval from the Food and Drug Administration to use naltrexone as an experimental treatment in alcoholics. In pilot studies, several patients reported a lack of enjoyment from drinking alcohol while taking naltrexone. Based on those observations, Chuck and his trainee Joe Volpicelli carried out the first double-blind, placebo-controlled trial of naltrexone in alcoholism. Male military veterans in an outpatient treatment program all received regular counseling and group therapy using the twelve-step methods of AA. In addition, however, they were also randomized to receive either 50 mg naltrexone daily or placebo. The dose was selected because it had previously been observed to block the high from heroin. Whether through sheer luck, amazing foresight, or both, the outcome that was chosen was not the traditional, which is to stay totally abstinent. Instead the thinking was that if naltrexone blocks the reward from alcohol, then maybe people would still have slips but in the absence of reward would not progress further and have a relapse to heavy drinking.

Despite the intensive behavioral treatment, 54 percent of patients receiving placebo relapsed to heavy drinking within three months. As we have seen, that result is fairly typical. In contrast, relapse occurred in only 23 percent of patients receiving naltrexone. When Stephanie O'Malley and her colleagues at Yale conducted a similar study in both male and female outpatients, they obtained very similar results. Both sets of results were published, back to back, in the same issue of a leading scientific journal in 1992.[26] As a result, naltrexone was approved for alcoholism treatment in 1994 under the name Revia.

More than thirty years after these seminal studies, and some fifty randomized controlled trials later, there is no question that naltrexone treatment has positive effects in alcohol addiction.[27] But the story of naltrexone is one that invites both a bottle half full and bottle half empty perspective. On one hand, the development of this medication was a groundbreaking discovery. For the first time there was solid evidence that alcohol addiction could be treated with a medication that acted on the brain. Once again, my instructor in medical school and many other skeptics were proven wrong. Importantly, in contrast to methadone, this was not simply about replacing the addictive substance with a medication that acted as a stabilizer while still having an abuse liability of its own. Naltrexone does not have any addictive potential. Because of this, and because its positive effects were obtained in combination with traditional behavioral treatments, one could have hoped that its use would become uncontroversial. On the other hand, once all the naltrexone studies were put together in a meta-analysis, the effect size was not very impressive. In fact, it was on the same order as the better behavioral treatments. And the large American COMBINE study suggested that if a good behavioral treatment was given, naltrexone possibly did not offer any additional benefit.[28] With a limited effect size, no major pharmaceutical company committed to marketing it, and unexpected resistance among many treatment providers to medications of any kind, naltrexone just did not catch on. For a long time its use remained a marginal phenomenon, largely confined to academic treatment centers. And even there, less than 5 percent of patients with an alcoholism diagnosis received a naltrexone prescription.

But those of us who did take up prescribing naltrexone noticed something quite interesting. A significant minority of naltrexone-treated patients seemed to improve dramatically. Many of those patients had for years not been able to touch alcohol without having a major relapse. They were, if you remember the quote from the Big Book of AA, "powerless against the first drink." Now, while on naltrexone, if they slipped, they did not seem to have much of a high and did not relapse to heavy drinking. This was indeed striking. Others, on the other hand, did not seem to show any response to the treatment at all. Sifting through the various naltrexone studies revealed that the characteristics of a naltrexone responder seemed to be that he was male and had a strong family history of alcoholism. Meanwhile, it had been reported that subjects with a family history of alcoholism had a significantly greater endorphin response to alcohol in the laboratory. This was at the time only possible to measure in plasma, but it could be speculated that a similar release occurred in the brain. A working hypothesis emerged from these findings. Perhaps alcohol activated endogenous opioid release in the brain, producing reward via some of the same pathways as heroin[29] and ultimately activating classical dopaminergic reward circuitry? This was appealing as a hypothesis. But for a long time it remained just that—a hypothesis.

So there was a crossroads. If patients seemed to respond differently to naltrexone treatment and the overall effect was modest, one possible response was to write off the treatment and move on. That is essentially what most of the field did. Of course, in the age of the sequenced human genome and emergence of personalized medicine, there was an alternative option. If patients seemed to respond differently to a medication, maybe that was because they were, fundamentally, different. In this case there was particular reason to pay attention to that possibility. In 1998 Mary Jeanne Kreek's group at the Rockefeller University in New York had reported that people differ in an important manner in the DNA code for the mu-opioid receptor, the target for naltrexone.[30] About 15–20 percent of white people had a variant of the receptor that seemed to respond differently to activation. Maybe this difference had something to do with medications targeting this receptor?

To test if these genetic differences could be related to the differences in naltrexone response, Chuck O'Brien and his colleague David Oslin set out to bring in DNA samples from people who had participated in three different naltrexone studies. Half the samples were missing. This was an "after-the-fact" analysis, of which geneticists are inherently suspicious. There were also other limitations. But if one was willing to look beyond those, the results seemed quite striking. It appeared that only a minority of patients—those with the less common receptor variant—had a benefit from naltrexone treatment. For them, on the other hand, the benefit seemed quite substantial. The remaining majority of patients did not seem to have any benefit at all. Once the pronounced effect obtained in the smaller responder group was mixed up with the lack of effect among the nonresponder majority, the average effect appeared small.[31]

These data seemed to potentially explain much of the naltrexone experience, but the results were controversial. Some analyses of other studies seemed to support the proposed pharmacogenetic effect; others did not. Some people welcomed the prospect of personalized treatment; others did not. When the Penn team submitted a grant application to fund a decisive, prospective study to answer the question, one anonymous grant reviewer wrote that "this could not be true; and even if it were, we would not want to know about it, because it would imply that not everyone is equally entitled to a treatment." And the biological mechanism that could explain how the different receptor variants influenced naltrexone responses continued to elude the field. The controversy continued.

Meanwhile, our lab had carried out a series of studies in rhesus monkeys that could be pointing to the underlying mechanism.[32] Following up on those findings, we were able to test Oslin and O'Brien's hypotheses in people. To figure out the role of the mu-opioid receptor gene variants, Vijay Ramchandani in our program recruited one group of social drinkers in whom both copies of the receptor gene were of the common variant. He also recruited another group, of equal size, in which all participants carried at least one copy of the unusual receptor gene variant.[33] We recruited only men because women do not seem to respond to alcohol with much of a brain reward system activation in the first place.[34] We gave our subjects a very precisely controlled alcohol infusion in the PET scanner so that in fifteen minutes they went from not having any alcohol in the blood to 80 mg/dl, the legal limit for driving in most states. As we infused alcohol, we were able to measure the amount of dopamine released in the brain reward circuitry. The results were striking. Only people who carried a copy of the less common gene variant responded to alcohol with a robust dopamine release.[35] These were exactly the people who in Oslin and O'Brien's analysis had seemed to respond to naltrexone.

The chain of events appeared quite clear. Just as Chuck O'Brien had hypothesized, alcohol must be releasing endogenous opioids. These then act on their mu-opioid receptors, ultimately activating the "final common pathway" of dopaminergic brain reward circuitry. This seemed to be happening predominantly, or perhaps exclusively, in people with a particular kind of genetic makeup, namely, those who carry the less common mu-opioid receptor gene variant. Obviously, if naltrexone intervenes into the cascade alcohol → endorphin release → dopamine release → reward, the medication can have an effect only in people in whom alcohol turns on this cascade. In others, there is simply nothing for naltrexone to work on.

Appealing though these results were, the proof that the gene variant actually *caused* the difference was still not watertight. Even if we just count genetic differences between people that are made up of one DNA letter exchanges, people differ from one another at more than three million places in the genetic code. Because of our origin as a species, and because of the way these differences have developed through our evolutionary history, these differences tend to travel in packs. What that means is that if you have a particular variant at a certain address in the genome, you are also more likely to carry a number of specific variants at nearby locations. So when we recruited people with the less common mu-receptor gene variant, we could, for all we knew, also have been recruiting people with some other variant that we did not even know about. That unknown variant could be causing the differences between people.

Normally this would be the end of the road. There is no way, in a human research subject, to determine if the differences we saw in the PET camera were really caused by the variant we thought caused them or some unknown neighbor. Working with my colleagues Wolfgang Sommer and Annika Thorsell, we therefore turned to genetically modified mice to address that final question. We spent several years making mouse lines in which we cut out the mouse mu-opioid receptor gene and replaced it with the human gene. We inserted the most common human gene version in one of the lines without any additional changes. In the other line, we started out with the same DNA code, but before inserting it into the mouse, we changed just one letter—the one that distinguishes the two different variants of the human receptor gene. When all this was done, we had mice that were genetically identical throughout the three billion letters of their genetic code except in the one place we wanted to probe. Working with Larry Parsons at the Scripps Research Institute in La Jolla, we were then able to directly measure the dopamine release in their reward circuitry when they received alcohol. Just like the people in our PET study, the mice with the less common gene variant released four times more dopamine.

Annika and Wolfgang, who by now run their own labs in Sweden and Germany, respectively, have since shown that these mice also consume more alcohol and have a much better response to naltrexone treatment. The story is remarkably consistent. The one-letter change in the genetic code has turned out to be critical. It seems that Chuck O'Brien had been right all along. By now a meta-analysis of clinical treatment studies confirms that carriers of the less common mu-opioid receptor gene variant are twice as likely to respond to naltrexone as patients without this variant.[36] The question is, what are we to do with these data in clinical practice? For another few years, we cannot yet count on every patient carrying his or her genome sequence on a card in a wallet. Neither can we yet expect the individual physician to order a lab test to determine the genetic makeup of a patient. But the days when a genetic profile will be available in clinical practice are not too far off. And until then we should remember that a good history may do a good enough job of identifying naltrexone-responsive patients. If someone is male, has a strong family history of alcoholism, and had a stimulant-like response from alcohol when first beginning to drink, chances are the patient will respond. There is little to lose from trying.

In a somewhat different way, the challenges to finding the right match between patient and medication are also illustrated by the other brain-acting medication that is approved for treatment of alcoholism. The U.S.

Food and Drug Administration approved acamprosate, marketed under the name Campral, as an alcoholism medication in 2004. It had been approved in France already in 1989, and in the rest of Europe over the following years. In 1996 two ambitious evaluations of acamprosate were carried out at a large number of European treatment centers and published in leading medical journals.[37] Together these studies included more than seven hundred patients. The participants had been treated for a year in one of the studies, and forty-eight weeks in the other. Subjects had then been followed up for an equal amount of time after the study medication was discontinued. Notably both studies focused on a different outcome from that of the original naltrexone studies, which measured the ability of the medication to prevent relapse to heavy drinking. The outcome chosen in the acamprosate studies was instead the traditional one: the ability to increase chances of sustained abstinence. That is clearly a more challenging treatment goal. In both studies from 1996, only a small proportion of placebo-treated patients—about 7 percent in one and 17 percent in the other—were continuously abstinent throughout the duration of the respective study. In both cases this proportion was approximately doubled when acamprosate was given, a set of results that were both highly statistically significant. What was particularly remarkable was that the beneficial effects of acamprosate were sustained during the follow-up period, when patients no longer received any medication.

Today meta-analyses support the efficacy of acamprosate to improve abstinence rates.[38] There is, however, an interesting complication to those data. The meta-analyses are dominated by studies carried out in Europe, because that is where most of the acamprosate research was done. You wouldn't think that would be all that important. After all, how different can a medication effect be, say, in England compared to New England? But something strange happened with acamprosate as it traveled across the Atlantic. A large study, with about six hundred participants, was carried out in twenty-one American treatment centers to support an approval of acamprosate as an alcoholism medication in the United States. When the results of that study were in, the acamprosate- and placebo-treated patients did not differ on the predefined outcome measure, the percentage of days patients were abstinent during the six-month-long trial. In some analyses there was some benefit to receiving acamprosate. For instance, among the two hundred or so people who entered the study with an explicit goal of achieving abstinence, the benefit was very clear. But these kinds of after-the-fact analyses, while often able to generate important new hypotheses, are typically not considered valid to directly support approval of a medication.[39] Then, a few years later, acamprosate was evaluated as part of the large COMBINE study mentioned previously, where naltrexone showed a modest but significant benefit.[40] Once again, no beneficial effect was found for acamprosate.

This seemed strange. The European studies were large, solid, and consistently positive. The American studies were large, solid, and consistently negative. What could possibly be going on? Although I cannot claim to have the definitive answer, I think it has by now become pretty clear that the effects of acamprosate differ from those of naltrexone in a fundamental way. For instance, if you give naltrexone to rats that self-administer alcohol, self-administration rates will consistently decrease, in any rat. That is what you would expect from a drug that in part blocks the rewarding, or reinforcing, effects of alcohol.[41] I still remember our disappointment when we first gave acamprosate to rats under the same conditions in my old lab in Stockholm. Nothing whatsoever happened to self-administration rates. But the results were very different when we first induced a prolonged state of physical alcohol dependence in our experimental animals. After we had done that, we let them come out of withdrawal and then sit on a shelf for three weeks. By that time the animals self-administered twice the amount of alcohol compared to animals without a history of dependence. Under those conditions, acamprosate brought down self-administration rates by half, reducing them to the levels of nondependent animals.[42] These and similar animal experiments suggested that for acamprosate to have an effect, long-term changes in brain function must be in place as a result of alcohol dependence.

With those data in mind, the European and American results make a lot more sense. The patients in the European studies typically had almost twice the alcoholism severity compared to those in the American trials. This is not because there is a European and an American version of alcoholism! It is simply a function of how studies recruit their participants on the two continents. All European countries have publicly funded health care, including addiction treatment centers. The standard approach to recruiting patients into a treatment study is therefore to go into the clinical population that seeks treatment at these centers and offer them a chance to participate. These participants tend to be more severely dependent, treatment-seeking, "real" alcoholics. In contrast, in the United States private health insurance, managed care, and liability issues make it difficult to access a regular clinical population for recruitment into a research study. So to a large extent investigators get their subjects by advertising in newspapers. That way they end up drawing from a population that tends to be socially more stable and in many cases perhaps would not have sought regular treatment. Those people tend to have less severe alcohol problems.

We still don't know the exact molecular mechanism with which acamprosate works, but these observations fit in well with the things we do know. As alcohol is taken acutely, it dampens the activity of glutamate, the main excitatory neurotransmitter of the brain. But during withdrawal there is a rebound, and glutamate activity goes into hyperdrive. That is why during withdrawal almost all brain systems appear hyperactive and hyperexcited— as an example, just test someone's knee-jerk reflex as he or she goes through alcohol withdrawal. Reflexes, of course, become hyperactive already at relatively modest withdrawal intensities. During severe withdrawal, excitability can become so pronounced that people go into delirium tremens or have seizures. Over time the excessive glutamatergic activity of acute alcohol withdrawal subsides and things calm down. But with repeated cycles of intoxication and withdrawal, brain function changes progressively, and there is more and more of a residual overactivity of glutamatergic nerve cells. Through mechanisms that are not yet well understood, this contributes to alcohol cravings and escalation of alcohol intake. Acamprosate can normalize this hyperactive glutamate transmission, as first shown in mice in a beautiful paper by Rainer Spanagel and his laboratory in Germany and then confirmed in patients with alcoholism by our own group.[43]

So the lessons from the acamprosate experience once again highlight the need for personalized treatment, tailored to characteristics of the individual patient. In the case of acamprosate, however, what seems most important is not the genetic makeup of the patient. Instead it is the history, and specifically alcoholism duration and severity. If patients with low severity of dependence are treated, we are unlikely to get clinically meaningful effects. Acamprosate seems primarily to be useful in patients with a high severity and long history of alcohol dependence. Although that may not sound as a fancy or modern as genetically determined personalized medicine, it is of course just as important.

I am convinced this is what the future looks like. For each new medication, we will need to carefully consider whether there are differences, genetic or otherwise, that make people more or less likely to respond. This will be particularly important in alcoholism because this is perhaps the most complex addiction, with many different brain systems engaged, and differentially so in different people. If we fail to understand these differences and don't target the right system in the right patient, we may fail to detect that a medication is promising in the clinical studies to begin with.

Also, we are not quite done with alcoholism medications yet. The three medications we have discussed so far—disulfiram, naltrexone, and acamprosate—are the ones currently approved by the Food and Drug Administration for treatment of alcohol dependence. So I guess they are the ones I can safely talk about without a risk of being sued. But there is more under way. In Europe nalmefene, a chemical relative of naltrexone but one that is safer to use in patients with liver damage, has recently been approved. Interestingly, it has been found effective using a targeted medication approach—taken only in anticipation of consuming alcohol, with the objective of preventing relapse to heavy drinking. That is the treatment approach I described in the vignette with my patient the track and field athlete earlier in the book. Although targeted treatment seems to contradict much of conventional wisdom about complete abstinence as the only worthwhile treatment goal, it may be able to help people who are not yet willing to endorse that kind of goal but are willing to start doing something about their drinking.

In addition, several other medications, although not approved for alcoholism treatment, have shown promising effects in alcoholism treatment studies. Some of these medications are already on the market, approved for other diseases. Perhaps best supported among them is the epilepsy medication topiramate, which in two large, independent, and well-designed studies were effective in reducing heavy drinking and also reduced the medical consequences of alcohol use.[44] Another very promising set of results was obtained with the muscle relaxant baclofen, which in an excellent study was found to be safe and effective for treatment of alcoholism in people with severe liver damage, who cannot be treated with naltrexone.[45] Neither topiramate nor baclofen is likely to receive approval as an alcoholism treatment, for purely commercial reasons. The costs associated with obtaining FDA approval for a new indication are considerable. Both baclofen and topiramate are old molecules; the baclofen patent expired in 1986, and the last patent for topiramate came to an end 2009. Generics have now long been available at low cost, and investing in approval of a new indication simply isn't commercially viable. With recent lawsuits, it is also unclear whether "off-label" prescription will be possible, even with the best possible scientific evidence supporting these medications. Ironically, perhaps the only hope that alcohol-dependent patients will benefit from the elegant science is therefore if someone develops molecules that are similar enough to these two to have the same effects, but different enough so that they can be patented and sold at premium price.

Beyond all the alcoholism medications I have described in this chapter, a host of additional experimental therapeutics are in various stages of evaluation. Some have reached clinical studies. Others have shown promise in animal experiments and are awaiting evaluation in humans. This rich landscape probably reflects the complex nature of alcoholism. There is never going to be a single magic bullet that will effectively treat all alcohol-addicted patients. Instead, improvements will be incremental, as each new medication is added to the armamentarium, and as we identify the patients most likely to respond to that medication. The multitude of medication candidates in alcoholism is not just a good thing. Considerable challenges are associated with sifting through all these medications. To give you an idea, even a minimalistic clinical study for alcoholism, with about 150 subjects and a duration of twelve weeks, costs about ten million dollars and takes a couple of years to carry out. Unless we can generate some interest from the pharmaceutical industry, there will be an increasing need for academia and government to step up to the plate if we are ever to bring any of the promising candidates to the patients who need them. But overall there is considerable promise that new medications will improve alcoholism treatment outcomes in the years to come. That is, if they are put to clinical use, of course.

This is going to be one of the shortest sections of the book. In it, I will discuss all the medications with a solid evidence base for other addictive disorders than those discussed so far—most important, addiction to cocaine, amphetamine, and other stimulants, as well as to cannabis.

There are none.

This is a sad state of affairs. These addictions are frequently associated with death and disease. Behavioral treatments are only modestly effective. In the years ahead, there is clearly important work to do for those who are trying to develop medications for these conditions.

It is in a way particularly sad and ironic that no effective medications for cocaine and other stimulant addictions have been discovered. The mesolimbic dopaminergic reward system has for decades now been the celebrity of addiction research. Cocaine and stimulants are the addictive drugs that most directly act on this system. You may remember the mechanism. Under normal, healthy conditions, dopamine that has just been released, once it has done its job at the receptor, is sucked back up into the nerve cell that released it, so that can be reused. This is done by a molecular pump called the dopamine transporter. Cocaine blocks the dopamine transporter, resulting in an abnormal accumulation of dopamine at the receptors. Amphetamine and its chemical relatives even make the transporter go into reverse gear, or invert it, so that it pumps out even more dopamine onto the receptors. The resulting dopamine levels that the receptors get exposed to can easily be tenfold higher than those that are present in the absence of drugs.

One would think that all the research on the role of dopamine in addiction, which over the decades has cost billions of dollars, would by now have resulted in the discovery of some medications able to counter the addictive effects of these drugs. It has not. Perhaps the dopamine system is simply so fundamental to goal-oriented, motivated behavior that it is not easy to intervene into its function without creating more problems than one is solving. With their dopamine receptors blocked, people easily become apathetic and unable to experience normal pleasures. And dopamine is of importance for other brain functions than motivation and reward as well. For instance, blockers of dopamine receptors, if dosed at high enough levels, will essentially stop all voluntary movement. Long-acting activators, the equivalents of methadone or a nicotine patch but for cocaine addicts, do not seem to work either—they all seem to have profound addictive potential of their own. Nor do partial activators, the equivalents of buprenorphine or varenicline. When one of those was tested in a study of amphetamine use, people used more, not less. I just don't know why that is.

Perhaps research focus will in the future need to shift to modulator systems that interact with the dopamine circuits rather than those circuits themselves. Or perhaps there are other approaches that I simply cannot think of, because if I could, the discovery would already have been made. But there is another, troubling possibility. Perhaps addictions to drugs that so directly intervene in the core of the brain's motivation and reward circuitry are just very difficult to treat. Perhaps there is no guarantee of success. Yes, there are a few potentially promising medications in early stages of evaluation. But I don't want to create too much hope. So far the track record is, to put it mildly, not encouraging. But I do hope this will change through the hard work of scientists pursuing novel treatments for these difficult-to-treat addictions.

18

PRAY IF YOU WISH, BUT PLEASE TAKE YOUR MEDS FIRST

THE WOMAN ACROSS my office table was visibly upset. She had asked to be discharged against medical advice, and her bags were already packed. Before sending her home, the attending physician alerted me to the situation, and I offered to meet with the patient. I guess listening to her concerns was a way of trying to show her respect. Maybe she would find the conversation helpful. Maybe there could be lessons for us to learn as well. I asked for the chart ahead of time and read up. This was an Ivy League–educated lawyer, in her early fifties. After years of heavy drinking that followed a traumatic divorce, she had worked hard to rebuild her life. By now she was back to work part time at a Washington, D.C., law firm and in a new relationship. But her financial situation was shaky. The part-time job did not provide health insurance, and without it there was no way she could afford residential treatment. When she relapsed, she contacted our program. Luckily the social worker who evaluated her on the phone was able to check all the right boxes. It seemed the caller was eligible for one of our ongoing research protocols. This was a study to test whether a new anti-stress medication could help anxious alcoholics reduce their urges for alcohol, so it seemed ideal. And participation, of course, came with the benefit of a free month of inpatient treatment at the Mark O. Hatfield Clinical

Research Center, the amazing research hospital located on the NIH campus in the Maryland suburbs.

After the phone screening, the patient was scheduled for admission and arrived as planned. The initial evaluation and consent process went fine, but it did not take many days on the unit before she began to have issues with some of the community rules. Now, maintaining the structure of everyday life on a treatment unit is challenging on the best of days. People come in with complicated problems, in different stages of withdrawal, and with very different backgrounds. They all need attention to different things, many of those very private in nature. Yet for a short time, all patients also become members of a small community. They can draw strength from one another, but there can also easily be frictions. That kind of community is hard enough to keep running smoothly in a regular treatment setting. Imagine, then, the challenges of combining that task with repeated blood sampling, psychological evaluations, brain scans, and other research procedures. Bringing all that together and still having a good treatment environment is complex beyond my imagination. I truly admire the dedicated nursing staff in our program that makes this work every single day, month after month. It is largely a mystery to me how they do it. But both the treatment and the research get done. And it seems that most of the time, there is the right balance between structure and a friendly, caring atmosphere. Conflicts rarely rise above whether someone just back from a research procedure should be allowed to turn on the television while other patients are still in a treatment group. And those conversations, too, tend to end with a joke and a smile.

This time was different, though. The issue was not one that was easy to joke away. The patient, an outspoken leftist liberal, was simply a nonbeliever. Not an "I don't attend any particular church, but I'm sure spirituality is good" type of nonbeliever; more of a "religion is the opium of the masses"[1] kind.

So here we were. Like most places, our treatment groups were shaped after the principles of "twelve-step facilitation." Although made more generic than the original, this is an approach to treatment that is firmly rooted in the Big Book of Alcoholics Anonymous,[2] all twelve steps of it. Famously written by William Griffith Wilson ("Bill W") and Dr. Robert Holbrook Smith ("Dr. Bob"), the Big Book may be under your radar if you have not been exposed to the addiction treatment scene. But as a treatment manual its popularity will surely never be surpassed. Since it was first published in 1939, it has sold over thirty million copies, making it one of the most widely disseminated books of all times, alongside the likes of the Harry Potter series and the Bible. All these years later, this is a book I personally still find to be amazing reading. It is earnest, brutally so at times, such as in the chapters "Bill's Story" and "Dr. Bob's Nightmare." It is, given that the better part of a century has passed since it was written, brilliantly insightful about many of the fundamentals of addiction. This is perhaps most striking in its framing of addiction as a disease, one that is chronic in nature and associated with changes that for life make most patients vulnerable to relapse. Hence the principle that "once an alcoholic, always an alcoholic," and the conclusion that only lifelong abstinence can lead to recovery.[3] Besides all the specifics, I find the Big Book quite heartwarming. After all, its fundamental concept is that by joining a fellowship, people can help one another overcome alcoholism and the adversity that comes from it. What is there not to like?

But at the same time, the book is clearly a product of its time. Just as an example, don't turn to it for a modern view on women and addiction. The first members were only men, and the most prominent notice of women was in a chapter entitled "To Wives." Likewise, the Big Book was obviously unable to reflect a modern scientific understanding of addiction as a brain disease or take into account evidence from controlled treatment studies. It was, after all, written long before either of those even got started. In fact, to put the roots of the AA movement in context, we need to understand the perception of alcoholism and its treatment in the early twentieth century. At the time this was a condition not only viewed as a moral failing but also thought to be largely hopeless. Beyond supportive care of acute complications such as delirium tremens, the medical profession had little to offer. William Silkworth, the New York physician who repeatedly cared for Bill Wilson and ultimately wrote the foreword to the Big Book, was way ahead of his time when he articulated a view of addiction as a disease. Over the course of successive admissions, he was able to convince Wilson that his drinking problem was not one that came from moral inferiority. Instead,

Wilson realized that he suffered from a disease, one that made him vulnerable to what we would today call the priming effects of the first drink, the loss of control that follows, and the consequences of the relapse to heavy drinking that results. But Silkworth had no naltrexone, varenicline, topiramate, or behavioral relapse prevention techniques to offer his patients. In fact, when he wrote the foreword, he was faced with a complete lack of effective medical treatments.

Because of the devastating natural history of alcoholism and the lack of effective medical treatments at the time, Silkworth and the founders of AA had to seek hope in something outside themselves, and outside professional treatment. Similar to countless men and women facing various kinds of adversity in prescientific times, they found it in a higher power. In the case of AA, this is a concept that should be understood very broadly. Compared to most organized religion, the Big Book and the AA movement as a whole are a marvel of tolerance and open-mindedness. They do not favor any specific congregation or religion, and they welcome everyone who wishes to join. But make no mistake: for AA, the key to successful recovery lies not primarily in understanding the addicted brain in scientific terms and then using that understanding to help the brain's owner recover control of his or her life. Instead the only hope for recovery is seen in admitting defeat and transcending the failings of the addicted brain by turning to the higher power. For those unfamiliar with them, let's take a look at the twelve steps of AA, which encapsulate this thinking and remain the basis for the movement.

1. We admitted we were powerless over alcohol—that our lives had become unmanageable.
2. Came to believe that a Power greater than ourselves could restore us to sanity.
3. Made a decision to turn our will and our lives over to the care of God as we understood Him.
4. Made a searching and fearless moral inventory of ourselves.
5. Admitted to God, to ourselves, and to another human being the exact nature of our wrongs.
6. Were entirely ready to have God remove all these defects of character.

7. Humbly asked Him to remove our shortcomings.

8. Made a list of all persons we had harmed, and became willing to make amends to them all.

9. Made direct amends to such people wherever possible, except when to do so would injure them or others.

10. Continued to take personal inventory and when we were wrong promptly admitted it.

11. Sought through prayer and meditation to improve our conscious contact with God, as we understood Him, praying only for knowledge of His will for us and the power to carry that out.

12. Having had a spiritual awakening as the result of these Steps, we tried to carry this message to alcoholics, and to practice these principles in all our affairs

One would be hard pressed to find any aspect of this message offensive. But it is also hard to escape its spiritual, rather than scientific, focus. More than half the steps directly speak of a god, a godlike power, or prayer. For starters, that is clearly not for everyone. But that is not necessarily a problem, as long as people for whom this is meaningful and appealing benefit from participating. The question is, then, how do we select those people, and what are those benefits? The answers to these two key questions need to be viewed in the context of a widespread American perception that twelve-step programs are the standard of addiction care.

It is frequently said that people who attend AA for a certain time and beyond do better than those who don't. The second edition of the Big Book, published in 1955, stated as a rule of thumb that among alcoholics who "really tried" to follow the AA program, "50% got sober at once and remained that way; 25% sobered up after some relapses, and among the remainder, those who stayed with Alcoholics Anonymous showed improvement." Surveys published by AA since then seem to be roughly in agreement with those numbers. This may sound appealing. But if we think back to the standards by which modern medicine evaluates interventions, things quickly become more complicated. As we have learned, the only way to really determine the effects of an intervention is to carry out a randomized, controlled trial:

a study in which participants are randomly allocated to the intervention we want to evaluate or an appropriate control condition. So counting what proportion of people who sign up for AA actually stay in AA does not tell us much. In fact, it has recently been recognized that just by deciding to enter a treatment or a clinical trial for alcoholism, people decrease their alcohol use by as much as two-thirds—whether they subsequently receive active medication or sugar pills.[4] So any specific treatment effects would have to show up as a significant difference between the control group and the active group, on top of the improvement in the controls. When it comes to behavioral treatments in general, it may also be a challenge to find the appropriate control condition. Randomization may not be easy. In the case of AA, for example, it would be very difficult to randomize people so that they either engage with the fellowship of AA or not. Absent that, we are left wondering if the numbers reported really represent an improvement over the natural history of the disease or over some alternative intervention.

Furthermore, even assuming that these outcomes are better compared to not participating, the surveys do not allow us to disentangle what is causing what. To what extent do outcomes that are reported actually reflect effects of AA participation? To what extent are they the result of the fact that people who are better able to stay sober in and of themselves are also more likely to stick with AA? "Really tried" has in the AA surveys often been interpreted as sticking with participation for at least ninety days. But analyzing the data that way brings up a classic problem that evidence-based medicine has had to deal with in all areas of clinical practice. This kind of "completer analysis" has a well-known source of error: it selects people who had inherently better chances of achieving good outcomes anyway. Imagine if you were treating cancer but included in your analysis only people who completed a one-year course of treatment. If people who did not get included had all dropped out because they had a particularly malignant form of the disease and were in fact dead by the one-year follow-up, the outcomes for those who remained in treatment for a year would look great! The same, of course, applies if people with particularly hard to treat addiction relapse within the first three months and drop out of AA participation.

It is well-known that a completer analysis routinely overestimates treatment effects or finds them where they are not really present. If we are evaluating a clinical treatment, there is therefore a known remedy for this problem. Every modern medication study is required to apply this remedy for the results to be considered valid. The FDA would never approve a new medication unless study outcomes had been evaluated that way. That standard is to carry out an "intent-to-treat" analysis in which anyone whoever got the first pill, or attended the first therapy session, is included. By that measure, AA's own surveys indicate that about half the people who start attending meetings drop out within three months. By the end of the first year, only 26 percent of the intent-to-treat population is still participating. That is very close to the classic relapse rates reported for most addictions, which are around 70 percent over twelve months.

Finally, even if we were able to detect beneficial effects of AA participation in a valid manner, it would be hard to know to what extent they are the result of following the twelve steps. There is no obvious way to distinguish that possibility from generic effects of being in a group of supportive people who share one's experience as well as one's goals, and who encourage one to stay sober. Maybe joining a chamber orchestra of recovering alcoholics, practicing Baroque music a couple times every week, and having a festive but alcohol-free meal together on the weekends would be just as good? That is how one of my hardest to treat patients, a university professor, finally achieved stable recovery. But I will never know what in that mix that did the trick. It would be difficult to demonstrate the specific influence of the chamber orchestra participation, the music that the group played, or the Sunday dinners. Or maybe the patient had just reached the point in life when he would have sobered up no matter what, and that in turn enabled him to join the chamber orchestra. Who knows? An individual life is an experiment run without controls.

With these observations in mind, it should not be entirely surprising to read the "Plain Language Summary" of a large meta-analysis published in 2006 by the International Cochrane Collaboration, the gold standard of evidence-based medicine:

The available experimental studies did not demonstrate the effectiveness of AA or other 12-step approaches in reducing alcohol use and achieving abstinence compared with other treatments, but there were . . . limitations with these studies. Furthermore, many different interventions were often compared in the same study and too many hypotheses were tested at the same time to identify factors which determine treatment success.[5]

All in all, this lack of reliable evidence for clinical benefits, obtained through scientifically valid methodology, would be devastating if we were evaluating a professional treatment. It would be worse still if patients or the taxpayer collective were being asked to pay a great deal for it. But neither the former nor the latter is the case. Enlightened AA members would be the first to point out that theirs is not a professional treatment that has as its objective to replace other treatment options. Instead it is simply a fellowship of addicts and recovering addicts who are willing to support each other in achieving and maintaining recovery. There is a mantra that has a lot truth to it: AA is everywhere, and it is free. As such, AA may really be outside the scientific medical paradigm. It does not lend itself well to the type of evaluation that is at the core of evidence-based medicine. In a sense, then, if we view the AA movement appropriately, the data may not be all that critical, as long as AA is not confused with professional treatment.

The bottom line for me is this: achieving recovery from addiction is a daunting task. For a long time, professional medical or behavioral treatments had essentially nothing effective to offer for this devastating disease. To date, treatments that have emerged are with a few exceptions only modestly effective.[6] Even as these treatments improve, people will continue to need support outside the professional treatment setting in order to live lives that are both worthwhile and free of alcohol and drugs. As long as we can work together, communities of people that vouch to provide one another support in staying sober and drug free surely should be a great complement to professional, evidence-based treatments. Perhaps the only valid criterion for whether these mutual-help groups are valuable is whether the people who participate in them feel that they are. When that is the case, we should encourage patients to seek them out. It is much like someone who is overweight, has developed type 2 diabetes, and decides to join a church that promotes a healthy lifestyle, or the Sierra Club and its hiking group. If the patient feels that this is helpful, then we should support him or her to stick with it, while at the same time tightly managing the metformin prescriptions and controlling blood sugar. Clearly AA is a major resource where countless patients find support for a drug-free life. It should be equally clear that, because of its spiritual focus, AA is not for everyone. Other options may be a better match. The same enlightened AA member who points out that AA is not a professional treatment would probably also agree with me in this: while the AA fellowship welcomes everyone with an addiction, it may not necessarily be *for* everyone with one.

So over my years in the field, I have taken a pragmatic approach to the tensions that may arise between medical treatments and AA participation. We, meaning the medical profession, do the best possible, science-based medical and psychological treatments currently available. We also work hard to develop new methods. At the same time, we happily introduce or reintroduce patients to AA, a resource we know many have found to be helpful in trying to achieve and maintain recovery. Some patients come back from their first AA meeting and describe an immediate feeling of having found a home. For many among our patients, with broken families, lost jobs, and lives filled with numerous challenges caused by their addictions, that is a big deal. Finding that kind of home may turn into a lifelong source of support. But other patients instinctively turn around in the doorway. There are many reasons why AA may not be for them. Or maybe they just do not feel like they belong, without being able to put their finger on why. That too has to be respected. In those cases we try to find other ways to support and manage long-term recovery. It is really that simple, at least in theory.

I have occasionally run into the typical problems that can come up in reconciling good medical management of patients with their participation in AA or other client groups. For instance, because lifelong abstinence is such a key tenet for AA, and because it is hard for laypeople to understand different effects of chemicals on the brain, many AA groups long viewed psychiatric medications with a great deal of skepticism. In those days it could happen that a patient I had finally been able to successfully treat for a devastating depression would be told by his AA sponsor to discontinue the medication. Sometimes I didn't even know about it until after the fact. In one case the way I found out was when a patient quickly worsened and attempted suicide. But I have realized that this perhaps wasn't primarily about AA. There is nothing in the twelve steps or in the Big Book that says you should not have evidence-based treatment for your depression. Except for the steps and the traditions through which members of the fellowship support one another in recovery, AA "does not wish to engage in any controversy" and "neither endorses nor opposes any causes."[7] No one speaks for "AA." The views of each AA group are influenced by the backgrounds, education, and attitudes of its members. As public awareness of mental health issues has improved in general, it has done so among members of most AA groups as well. The best approach to these controversies has been to offer patients and their families solid information and invite them to bring their AA sponsors into the conversation. I am sure there are AA groups where these are still controversial issues. I am equally sure there are not nearly as many of those groups as there were when I started in the field.[8]

So where did things break down with our lawyer? As I said, the spiritual tone of the twelve-step facilitation group did not sit well with her. Understandably, as a convinced atheist, she would have none of the higher-power stuff. She asked for other options. In those days we didn't have any. She asked to not participate. Some of our staff told her she had to because that was the community rule, and if she didn't participate, others would soon stay away too. She tried, grudgingly, only to discover that the next group was held by the hospital pastor, who led it in prayer. After that things were beyond repair. The patient was not only a nonbeliever, she was also a fiercely independent person. As such, she did not respond well to having something imposed on her that was so contrary to her core beliefs. As a lawyer, she could not comprehend how a government agency could compel people to participate in what amounted to religious activities. As I listened to her account, I could see her point. I acknowledged as much, but without making excuses, I also tried to explain. Some of our staff were former alcoholics themselves. Although they had to be many years sober to work for us, they brought with them the experience of once having had support in their own recovery through AA, where they remained active members. Yes, it was unacceptable to impose their beliefs on patients, but it really was well intentioned. They just wanted for our patients what had been helpful to themselves.

By the end of our meeting, which lasted almost an hour, I was convinced we had both learned something. I offered to see the patient for a couple of follow-up appointments. She considered my offer of a naltrexone prescription but decided to try and stay sober by sheer power of will. I suspect that by then she may well have succeeded out of pure spite. I let her know I hoped it would work out, but also that she was welcome back if it didn't. At least it felt like we had worked out the issues that had upset her. After she left I gathered my staff and reinforced the principles I have outlined above. I charged them with creating a better distinction between what we do as medical professionals and what we support our patients in doing as self-help. I also charged the staff with developing alternative behavioral treatment options to the twelve-step facilitation groups so that all patients would have choices available to them that they could feel comfortable with. With that I thought things had been resolved in a way that had offered us all opportunities to grow.

A couple of weeks later, we learned that the NIH leadership had received a letter from someone in Congress regarding our treatment program. As we waited to hear about its content and discussed it with our institute director, I was puzzled. It clearly seemed likely that this would have to do with the recent incident. We had really never had anyone else be all that unhappy with the program. I had parted ways with the patient on a friendly note, convinced that she felt her concerns had been adequately addressed. Had I been so wrong? Was I becoming an insensitive bureaucrat, so that my clinical intuition was beginning to fail me? Finally, my boss and I arrived on Capitol Hill, to be heard by a couple of congressional staffers. As the first questions were asked, we looked at each other. This just didn't make sense. Then, gradually, we learned about the content of the letter. I will never forget my feeling of shock and disbelief. The complaint had not come from the patient. It had come from one of my nurses, a recovering alcoholic, AA member, and sponsor to a congressional staffer. The complaint was that under my leadership, our program, part of a U.S. government agency, had

turned against AA. This was unacceptable. The old routines were to be rein-
stated immediately, or else our institute would be made to feel the consequences during the upcoming appropriation process.

I was getting ready to argue. I was considering resigning. Fortunately
my boss helped me get over it. A wonderful internist, he had grown up in
Hungary and somehow always managed to cope with madness by cracking
a socialist era joke. We found a compromise solution, emotions cooled off,
and we were able to stay focused on our mission. These are not easy issues,
nor was this the first time they were debated. Already in 1999, the U.S.
Court of Appeals for the Second Circuit ruled that an atheist drunk driver's
constitutional rights were violated when he was forced, as a condition of
probation, to participate in a "religion-tinged Alcoholics Anonymous program." This triggered a fair amount of debate within the AA community.
Although there were clearly two sides to the debate, many AA members
felt that forcing people to participate runs counter to the core idea of AA
the way they know it: a voluntary fellowship of people intent on supporting
each other in recovery. I agree and in fact can't see how any other position
could be defensible. And I can't see how advising patients to discontinue or
avoid medications their doctor has recommended based on solid evidence
can be defensible either. I hope that these are marginal phenomena or will
become so with time. Meanwhile, I will continue to advise patients to try
out AA and see if it is for them. My responsibility as a physician will remain
to make sure patients get the best treatment data support, whether they feel
spirituality should be part of their recovery or not.

The Willmar Hospital Farm for Inebriates was originally built in 1907. It
is located in a small town in Minnesota, about a hundred miles west of
Minneapolis, in a community that to this day has a population of less than
twenty thousand. When Hospital Farm started, it had all of fifty beds. Over
subsequent years it went through a series of expansions and name changes.
Ten years after first opening its doors, it became the Asylum for the Insane
at Willmar but continued to provide care for addicts. Its origins and history parallel those of many institutions from that era, including the mental hospital back in Europe where I took my first steps along the way to

becoming a psychiatrist. Today, in the age of community-based mental health, it is easy to be harshly critical of those institutions. A reading of their history certainly makes one appreciate the progress made since those days. Asylums were once, into the late nineteenth century, simply prisons for the insane. They did not offer treatment, because there was none. Instead they practiced incarceration and restraint. Patients were caged, shackled, or put into straitjackets to prevent them from being violent to themselves or others or destroying property. Willmar was built in a time when new ideas about treatment of people who are mentally ill were beginning to emerge. The German physician Emil Kraepelin, the father of modern psychiatry, had published his major work, *Compendium der Psychiatrie*, in 1883. In it he argued that psychiatry is a branch of medicine and should be based on careful observation, just like the other natural sciences. There was a new emphasis on diagnosis of specific conditions, and the range of treatments started to expand. Restraints began being viewed as cruel and unnecessary. But it is easy to forget that much of the real progress was made possible only by the arrival, from the 1950s and on, of modern psychiatric medications. Only then did it for instance become possible to discharge chronically psychotic patients into the community. And as we know, it is to this day a considerable challenge to provide enough support for people with serious psychiatric conditions to live and function outside institutions.

Dan Anderson, a clinical psychologist by training, started at Willmar in 1951. As already mentioned, alcoholism was at the time widely viewed as a moral failing. Even as views of other mental disorders started to evolve closer to what we today would consider modern and ethically acceptable, there continued to be little sympathy in the community for the plight of those who suffered from addiction. The disorganized behaviors, the hallucinations, and the delusions of people with chronic psychoses started being viewed as specific symptoms of diseases that patients suffered from through no fault of their own. In contrast, people with addictive disorders were thought to have brought the adversities facing them upon themselves. Even at the asylum, the inebriates were "at the bottom of the patient pecking order," Anderson is quoted saying in an interview. "Everyone looked down on them, including the community, hospital staff, and even our mentally ill patients. The inebriates had a lower status than the schizophrenics and the manic depressives, or even the kleptomaniacs or pedophiles." Accounts from those days describe how Anderson, supported by Willmar's superintendent Nelson Bradley, set out on a mission to humanize alcoholism treatment and "transform treatment wards from snake pits into places where alcoholics and addicts could retain their dignity." Emphasizing that alcoholics are affected by their disease in ways that are medical, mental, and spiritual, Anderson made the twelve steps of AA the foundation of a new, "multiphasic" approach to addiction treatment, one that was interdisciplinary and attempted to integrate the different facets of the disease.

Based on these principles, Anderson's model was first developed at Willmar but continued to evolve to maturity at a location about 140 miles to the east, in Center City, Minnesota. This was the location of a farmhouse by a lake, donated by a benefactor in 1949, where things were started off by a staff of three, operating a guest house for alcoholics, with a daily headcount of less than ten. The guest house was not a treatment institution in any traditional sense of the word. The accounts of those days say that there were only a few set elements of daily life, and those would not typically be viewed as professional treatment. The guests were "simply required to behave responsibly, attend lectures on the twelve steps of AA, talk with the other patients, make their beds, and stay sober." Although this may not sound all that significant, these were the rather humble beginnings of the Hazelden Foundation, and what ultimately became the Minnesota Model. Fully developed through the 1960s, this model spread through the United States and the world in the 1980s and became that most widespread model for addiction treatment worldwide. Well-known addiction treatment centers, including institutions such as the Mayo Clinic and the Betty Ford Center, are patterned after the Hazelden model of care and in fact had help from Anderson and his coworkers in starting up their work. Anderson moved from Willmar to Hazelden full time in 1961 and remained active there until his death in 2003. He first was vice president, then president, and then president emeritus and is essentially the founder and the main architect of the Minnesota Model.

Today Hazelden occupies a unique center spot in the addiction treatment world, in particular in the United States. It has grown into a large treatment center at its original location, with satellites in ten locations across the country, a graduate school, a publishing house, and a research center. From 1996 the Butler Center for Research at Hazelden has given out an annual award in Dan Anderson's name. I had of course heard a lot about Hazelden through my years in addiction medicine, but when I received the Anderson Award in 2008 and started reading up, I found that my knowledge about the foundation and its history was nevertheless rather limited. As pleased on behalf of our whole research team as I was, I probably did not fully appreciate the significance. Here was an institution at the heart of the twelve-step tradition, actively welcoming and supporting the advances of modern addiction science. Among prior recipients were people I greatly admire. One of them was Stephanie O'Malley of Yale University, codiscoverer of naltrexone treatment for alcoholism, which, as I have indicated, remains controversial to this day with many twelve-step-based treatment programs. Another was Reid Hester from University of New Mexico, coauthor of the book on evidence-based addiction treatment that for me personally had once been an eye-opener, and that had many inconvenient truths to tell the field.

Indeed, the research that had earned us the award seemed quite removed from the core elements of the treatment traditions from which the Minnesota Model has grown. In a paper published in the journal *Science*, we had gone from a genetically modified mouse model to an experimental study in patients with alcohol addiction and made findings that could possibly represent the discovery of a new alcoholism medication. The emphasis, of course, should be the word "could." When it comes to diseases of the central nervous system, no matter how good things look at the early stages, only a very small fraction of new medications pan out in the long run. The brain and its behavioral disorders just seem to be difficult targets. After a golden era that culminated around the time of the introduction of depression medications Prozac and Cymbalta and the antipsychotic Clozaril, successes have been few and far between. Because of low return on investment, major pharmaceutical companies have over the past years pulled out from psychiatric disorders one by one. In addictive disorders, their interest had not been all that great to begin with.

With all the caveats, our findings did look quite promising. Mice with the gene for a particular neurotransmitter receptor knocked out did not escalate their alcohol consumption over time the way normal control mice did. They also seemed to have lost their reward from alcohol. In parallel, in collaboration with my longtime friend Don Gehlert and his colleagues at Eli Lilly, we studied an experimental drug that blocks the same receptor. We admitted patients with alcohol addiction to our research unit at the NIH Clinical Center and quickly got them either on the medication, a neurokinin 1 (NK1) receptor blocker, or sugar pills. As is standard in modern medication trials, neither the patient nor the research team knew who received the respective treatment. Once the study was over and we broke the blind, the results were clear. Participants who had received active treatment reported feeling better overall. A couple of weeks into treatment, we had exposed them to an experiment trying to mimic a situation that provokes relapse in the real world. Participants were exposed to a social stressor and then were asked to handle and sniff their favorite alcoholic beverage. They could not drink, but we let them rate how much they craved alcohol, and we were also able to simultaneously measure their stress hormones. Participants who had received the medication reported a reduction in craving and had markedly lower levels of the main human stress hormone, cortisol.

But it was the brain-imaging data that convinced me we may actually be on to something important. Together with a team headed by my colleague Dan Hommer, a fellow psychiatrist and the person from whom I have learned much of what I know about brain imaging, we studied the effects of the new medication on brain responses to positive and negative emotional stimuli. Dan and his group had previously shown that the brains of alcoholics overreact to negative emotional pictures, right in the brain areas known to process negative emotions. Teaming up with Dan's group, we saw the same highly reactive emotional responses in our placebo-treated study subjects. In contrast, patients treated with the experimental drug did not respond with any such activation. That was exactly what we had hypothesized and hoped for.

Another, unexpected finding was possibly even more compelling. Countless patients have described how, after many years of drinking, normally pleasurable experiences become gray and indifferent in the absence of alcohol. Although somewhat speculative, I think that the signature of this phenomenon was visible in our fMRI maps of the brain. Normally, pleasant visual stimuli are able to activate a network of reward-related brain structures. After many years of alcoholism, that activation was lowered or absent in our placebo-treated study participants, a finding consistent with several studies now available to show that reward responses in alcoholics fade over time. In contrast, these responses were restored in participants who had received active medication for a couple of weeks. Between the two findings described here, of down-regulated reactivity to negative stimuli and restored reactivity to pleasant images, we were most likely looking at the brain signature of a drug that made our subjects feel better and removed their incentives for resumption of alcohol use. This was perhaps a medication that, if it ever made it to the market, patients would actually want to take.

I was to receive the Anderson Award at the annual conference for the National Association of Addiction Treatment Providers in Florida. Carlton Erickson from the University of Texas-Austin, a member of the award committee and an expert on communicating the science of addiction to laypeople, had kindly provided me with comments and suggestions to tailor the talk to the intended audience. With his help I worked hard to avoid the two most common traps that a passionate scientist can fall into on an occasion like this. First, I tried to zoom out from our own research and provide as much as possible of the big picture of developing medications for alcoholism. When talking about the specifics of the things we do, I tried to put them in that broader context. Second, I cut out as many nonessential technical details as I possibly could.

But perhaps most important, I tried to address an issue I anticipated would come up. I knew that the vast majority of treatment providers in the United States are fundamentally committed to the twelve-step model. I also knew that most places, that remains associated with widespread skepticism against the use of medications for treatment of addictive disorders. Given my view of what is needed in the field of addiction, and what kind of research I do, it seemed clear that this topic needed to be addressed. I tried to do so in a thoughtful rather than provocative fashion. Still, as the conference neared, I had nightmares about people getting up to yell at me or leaving the room. But it turned out I could have saved myself the worry. May 2009 came, and I went to Florida. I recall a very kind introduction, and a nice crystal plaque being handed over. The talk went all right, but I have done enough of these to pick up the atmosphere in the room. It was clear that I was somehow unable to quite engage my audience. Afterward there were some of the predictable questions—whether medications weren't in fact only "crutches," stood in the way of "true" recovery, and the like. But the theme was not broadly picked up, and then people dropped off. By the time we got to the luncheon, it seemed quite clear that my one-hour lecture was a sideshow. I was puzzled. Clearly there was something here I was missing. I strolled between posters, and they seemed more like a trade show than a scientific meeting.

At the luncheon, when people got up and talked about their programs, it struck me how often success was presented in financial terms. I was seated next to Mark Mishek, at the time less than a year into his job as the new president and CEO of Hazelden. During the course of the conversation, he struck me as a sensible and nice man. Prior to Hazelden he had spent five years successfully running a major hospital in St. Paul, clearly no mean feat. We had a pleasant and interesting conversation. I was of course curious about Hazelden in general, but also specifically about their use of medications. Mark confirmed that only a very small percentage of people leaving their treatment did so with a prescription for one of the approved alcoholism medications. But he also spoke about their work on increasing that share. And he told me that Hazelden was beginning to work with David Oslin, a researcher at University of Pennsylvania, to study the role of genetics for the response to naltrexone. That really was on the cutting edge of science and pointed to the potential for personalized treatment. The study did happen,[9] with support from a donation received by Hazelden. All in all, this was a conversation very different in tone from what I was hearing in general at the meeting, and one from which I came away quite encouraged. But I could not figure out how to put the pieces together. How did this balanced, sensible, evidence-oriented man's vision rhyme with my other impressions of the treatment landscape—the resistance to any use of medications, the public brushing aside of scientific evidence that supports their use, such as I had seen by the chair of Betty Ford Center just a year earlier on CNN?

Two years later I had finally decided to write this book. Presenting the science was going to be challenging enough, but that is after all my job. What I knew I needed help to understand was the gap between what science tells us about addiction and its treatment, on one hand, and the industry that seems to provide expensive treatments that have little if any support from evidence, on the other. As I started thinking about whom to turn to, Mark Mishek was the first person who came to mind. I sent him an e-mail: Could we please schedule a phone call? Once we got on the phone, I tried to explain my ideas, at that time probably not very well articulated. Mark listened patiently. Then he responded, in not too many words, but in a way that made it clear he not only understood but had been thinking about many of the same things. I explained that it was hard for me to get a real feel for the issues on the ground without experiencing the treatment environment firsthand. Could I please come to Hazelden, spend a week, talk to people, and learn? Mark put me in touch with Valerie Slaymaker, a clinical psychologist and researcher who serves as provost of Hazelden's Graduate School of Addiction Studies. Training graduate-level addiction counselors is one of the many ways in which Hazelden has for a long time exerted a major influence on the world of addiction treatment in the United States and beyond. Valerie's interests include addictions treatment research and the implementation of evidence-based practices into clinical programming. She seemed ideally positioned for what I had in mind.

It took nine months to find the right time, but finally we were able to schedule a visit, for which Valerie and her colleagues put together a program.

I leave the simple hotel after an early breakfast. The hotel is located across the state line, in Wisconsin. As I cross the St. Croix River into Minnesota and start the climb up onto the plain, the landscape is glorious. The main road to Center City is closed for repairs, sending me off looking for county road 37 from Taylors Falls. It is a clear day late in September. The morning air, cool and fresh after the cold night, is radiant in the low sunlight. A veil of thin fog is rising from the fields as the soil wakes up, gently brought to life by the sun. The color palette surrounding me ranges from brown earth tones to the gold nuances of the crops, which, being a city boy, I don't even have names for. Straight roads cut through huge squares and rectangles of fields, looking as if they lead all the way to the horizon. Their straight lines make me wish I could just keep driving for hours, to see where the road might take me. I drive past ruminating cows, unperturbed by the passing stranger and his car. Over it all, a pale blue sky is arched like an endless cupola. On a day like this, it is hard to imagine that winter and snow are only weeks away.

When I arrive at my destination, the first thing that strikes me is the timeless quality of the buildings, and their harmony with the country-side. As I will learn later, the original farm house by the lake, the Old Lodge, was torn down to accommodate an expansion. Only the library that once belonged to Hazel Thompson, the woman after whom Hazelden is named, was preserved, as part of a new building. The place now has more than 150 beds, and close to two thousand people come through here each year with hopes of a new beginning. Then there are the graduate school, the research center, the retreat center, and more. It is clear from the park-ing lots, the signs, and the maps posted on the street corners that the cam-pus is huge. Yet at the same time it is as if the architects had tried to make the structures part of the landscape. The buildings on the gentle slopes have walls with the same color palette as the surroundings. The architec-ture reminds me a bit of Scandinavia, with brick walls that may not take on the elements head on but are made to resist them. Indoor walkways connect the buildings, ready to provide safe passage on a less friendly day. Half the people have names like Anderson, Carlson, or something of that nature. I try to joke with one of the women, the program director on the male Shoemaker Unit where I have my client immersion. "If it weren't for that-and-that letter in the spelling of your last name, you could be taken for a Norwegian, too." She smiles a wry smile. Yes, her husband's father did change the spelling. Yes, his family was from Norway, hers from Sweden. But she'd rather talk about the unit she runs, and the people who come through it.

I am an awkward participant in the groups. Without the professional role as a physician or a scientist to hide behind, I am lost in any group of more than three people, anywhere. Here I'm in a group with people who a week ago had never met yet now share stories so personal that they hurt just listening to. Is this about opening up and reflecting, despite the pain that may cause? Is it about seeking the support of others in the group, getting their help to deal with issues that weigh on these lives? Or is it about a moment's attention that in fact trivializes those same issues, making them into a kind of fleeting reality TV, before life goes on, unchanged? From what I see during my brief time here, for the most part it is definitely about the former. Occasionally, I'm afraid, the latter. Either way, the world of addicts I know, filled with urgency, disease, dirt, remorse, and lost hopes, seems far away. I guess in a way it really is. Not absent, just held at a distance, one that in part is simply physical. I learn that when his life finally came apart one day, one of the clients took a taxi here from the East Coast, on the inspiration of the moment. His trip must have been as stunning in terms of physical distance as it was in terms of contrast. He left chaos and arrived at a highly orderly daily routine.

Much of the time there is an edgy humor to this ordered existence. The unit has a rotating function as "pigmaster," and those who don't keep this temporary home clean and tidy get cited on the piglist. In the group session, once the piglist is dealt with, one of the clients, a thin, dark young man gets up and talks about life as a heroin addict on the streets of New York City. The brutality of the tale first seems surreal in these peaceful surroundings. Then, all of a sudden, an exchange starts between the young man and one of the middle-aged alcoholics and quickly comes to a flashpoint. The counselor is masterful in making sure the two men are both heard yet neither of them is hurt or diminished. When the group is over, I am all of a sudden part of a circle of men embracing each other and shouting out the battle cry of the Shoemaker Unit. I try to let go of feeling awkward and join them but succeed only in part. Instead the real meeting happens elsewhere. I join the clients for lunch in the cafeteria. This is one of my nightmares ever since I was a child—eating with strangers, stiffening up, never knowing what to say. To break the ice, I make a quiet comment about just that. A big, blond local farm boy, quiet until now, responds. It quickly becomes clear that he knows exactly what I am talking about, only on a different level. He talks of a glass bubble that surrounded him in high school. About trying it all, starting with meth, just to break out of it for a moment. About finally finding his best friend, alcohol, and how life spiraled down from there. Within minutes a circle of strangers is ever so briefly transformed into a circle of . . . what? Fellow humans, I guess.

During the course of the week, many people open their doors for me without asking for anything in return. From those people I learn as much as I had ever hoped and more. I learn how, after somewhat shaky beginnings of the retreat for professionals with alcoholism at the Old Lodge,[10] Pat Butler, a local businessman with alcoholism in the family, became the president and put the foundation on a sound financial footing. I learn how Hazelden in the 1960s, with Dan Anderson as the main architect, moved beyond a pure, traditional twelve-step approach, to make treatment multidisciplinary, over the years adding psychological and psychiatric services. From Dan Frigo, now dean of Hazelden's graduate school, I learn about the great expansion of the Minnesota Model in the 1980s. In those days, he tells me, he worked for a company, one of many that could be hired on a consulting basis to establish treatment facilities, much like how some builders put up standard home designs wherever they go. Most of those treatment programs were purely commercial. None of them were part of Hazelden, which remains a nonprofit foundation. I learn that in 2006, more than two years before I first met Mark Mishek, Hazelden started offering anticraving medications such as naltrexone, and how, from those slow beginnings, about 40 percent of alcohol dependent patients by now leave the program with a prescription for one of these medications. That, I note, is about tenfold better than typically happens in specialized addiction medicine services elsewhere. We also talk about preparations for introducing at least limited duration of buprenorphine maintenance into treatment of opioid addiction, despite the controversy that is likely to provoke in the AA community, because that is what the data support, and because it is unbearable to see patients die in the absence of that treatment. Since my visit, that program has indeed been implemented.

Some things I had been only vaguely aware of become clearer to me. When I first encountered the Minnesota Model, at the time it was imported to Europe around the late 1980s, I noticed that it quickly became oddly controversial. At the time I guess I didn't pay attention to the details. The impression was that big businesses were all of a sudden willing to pay considerable amounts of money to have key employees treated for addiction, in a way they had never before, but also one that did not entirely make clinical sense to me. The treatment was expensive and offered little in the way of continued management after the pricy month of residential treatment. Combine these two features, and too often an expectation of a "cure" was created, setting the scene for disappointment and cynicism. Meanwhile, social workers and addiction counselors rebelled against the treatment, in ways that did not always seem entirely rational either. None of this made much sense to me at the time, but I was too busy in the lab and elsewhere to learn more. In retrospect, I understand better. For starters, the spiritual tone of the foundation for the Minnesota Model did not go over well in Europe, which is increasingly secular. Combine that with the aggressively commercial pitch, and you can count on conjuring images of mega-church evangelists that enrich themselves at the expense of people who are gullible at best, and vulnerable at worst. That is a brew toxic enough to trigger all the resentment a secular, liberal intellectual is capable of.

Except not much of that really seems very relevant to what I encounter during my visit in Center City. Like any place, Hazelden has to pay the bills. A consequence of going from a bare-bones AA retreat at the Old Lodge to making treatment increasingly comprehensive is obviously that those bills increase. Just the modern medical detoxification unit, where newly arrived clients start out for as many days as they need to, is quite costly to operate. So are the psychiatric consult function and other components of the comprehensive, multidisciplinary treatment. Yet this is unmistakably a nonprofit. When I try to be penetrating with my questions, people instead join me in expressing concerns about how difficult it is to fund addiction treatment, anywhere. To a large extent, this is no different from the challenges confronting anyone attempting to provide health care to people without much in the way of resources. Except in this case, there is not a powerful medical profession aligned with those needs.

I spend some time with Stacy Weaver, the supervisor for the financial case manager group, and one of her coworkers. From them I learn about the battles they frequently fight on behalf of clients with insurance companies but also about the contracts they have over time been able to negotiate with some of the major insurers.[11] In the course of those conversations, we touch on other places that offer treatment, don't take insurance, and openly cater to a clientele of means only. The Hazelden staff don't expressly criticize those places, but they make a point of showing me how hard they try to do things differently. I learn about the partial stipends that a proportion of Hazelden's revenue is used for to help clients offset treatment cost. I learn that a couple of beds are always available for free to county residents, as an expression of gratitude for the support of the local community. We talk about efforts to support parity laws and in other ways advance an agenda of addressing the needs of people with addictions. We talk about the need, meanwhile, to develop less costly treatment options so that more people can have access to treatment. I bring up the need I see to create a continuum of care, one that is built on a recognition that addiction is a chronic, relapsing disorder. No one objects—the issue is high on the agenda—but they point out the shortage of treatment resources when clients return to their communities. There is a fun discussion about opportunities for creating online recovery management tools that in part can help fill this gap and provide support for a long time at a low cost. I get a fascinating look at a program that is being piloted.

I know people who care, and who know their stuff, when I see them. These are good people. Few of them talk about it, but in meeting them, a reference here or a statement there, made in passing, indicates to me that many of those I talk to know the hardships of addiction firsthand. They know how brittle the ice can be on which we walk through life. In most of the conversations I have, there is humility that perhaps has its roots in that fact. On a beautiful autumn day in Minnesota, it is easy to take all this in and be immersed in the serenity of the Hazelden campus. I suppose that is in part its purpose. It is easy to see how this environment fulfills the promise of creating a place to rebuild and give a feeling of dignity to people who were once at the bottom of the totem pole, even at the asylum in Willmar. Today, as I learn, this combines with a considerable degree of openness to science and an ongoing change in practice, driven by scientific data. I discover more common ground than I had perhaps expected, and the feeling is quite powerful. Yet for all the beauty, dignity, generosity, and openness I encounter, my job is to ask the hard questions. I will try to articulate those in the final chapter.

19

THE JOURNEY AHEAD

T HE AMOUNT OF pain, suffering, and cost to society caused by addictive disorders is beyond imagination. I hope that the patient vignettes I have sketched from my years of practice have helped get past the statistics and put faces of real people on the numbers. The consequences of addiction affect patients, their families, and their communities. As if that were not bad enough, they are frequently passed on to future generations, through violence, disrupted families, and poverty. Given the disease and economic burden to people and society associated with addictive disorders, the resources devoted to addressing these conditions are woefully inadequate. The disparity is certainly striking at the level of research as well. Just as an example, the U.S. government alcohol research institute for which I work receives approximately one-tenth of the funding devoted to cancer research. It is clear that this does not reflect the relationship between the disease burdens caused by the respective disease groups. But the disparity is even greater at the level of treatment. Patients with devastating addictions lack access to treatments that could help them. This is driven both by financial factors and by attitudes. I hope to have made clear how these two sets of factors are related to each other. A large part of the public continues to view addictive disorders as moral defects rather than treatable medical conditions and continues to elect policy makers who share their views.

I further hope to have made the case that addiction needs to be viewed as a chronic relapsing disorder, not unlike many other medical conditions. In the case of type 2 diabetes, numerous genetic factors interact with lifestyle, resulting in a disrupted ability to regulate blood sugar. In the case of addiction, numerous genetic factors interact with lifestyle, resulting in disrupted behavioral control and self-regulation of drug use. Several important conclusions arise from this insight. One is that, for now at least, any promise of "cure" is somewhere between naïve and dishonest, depending on who makes it and why. But it is equally true that these chronic relapsing disorders can now be managed so that most people with such disorders can decrease their risk for relapse, allowing them to live productive, good lives. Much of this opportunity is created by scientific advances in the understanding of what factors trigger relapse, as well as the development of psychological and pharmacological approaches that minimize relapse risk. Simply by providing patients with treatments that are based on these advances and are supported by scientific evidence, we would dramatically reduce death, disease, and cost from addiction. Among the treatments that should be provided but are not, relapse-prevention techniques based on methods of cognitive-behavioral therapy have well-documented, albeit modest, effects across the entire spectrum of addictive disorders. So do several medications, such as naltrexone for alcoholism and methadone and buprenorphine for opioid addiction. Several additional medications with promising data to support them already are on the horizon.

The past half century has made tremendous inroads toward understanding the brain basis of complex behaviors. Among those advances, the neuroscience of addiction is perhaps one of the most amazing success stories. These advances have only recently started to inform efforts to develop new treatments. But in addition to the already documented mechanisms, numerous mechanisms whose contribution to various aspects of addiction we are beginning to understand offer a hope of novel treatments. We need to be cautious. There is no way to be certain that this promise of new, science-based treatments will materialize. There are many reasons why it might not. If the brain changes triggered by addiction are largely structural rather than functional, then medications may simply not be able to set things right. But I am modestly hopeful. This is in large part because, even when structural changes have occurred, the human brain and the behaviors it produces show a tremendous degree of plasticity and potential for change. We already have several medications that can positively influence the course of an addictive disorder by interacting with systems that mediate rewarding properties of drugs. I am hopeful that new molecules that target stress systems, or the "dark side of addiction," will soon offer additional treatment options. And then there is the potential for targeting the impairment in decision making that is part of addiction and contributes to maintaining it. Although this may seem harder to achieve with medications, it has been possible to improve decision making and cognition in disorders such as ADHD. So there is no reason to exclude the possibility that it may be successful in addiction as well.

Beyond these advances, a more fundamental issue lies ahead of us. Is every person with an addiction forever bound to struggle with the consequences of brain function changes that underlie their addicted state? Will treatments need to be given for decades or a lifetime to keep countering those changes? If a person, for instance, has become prone to relapse when faced with stress, is that person forever going to be in need of treatments that dampen their sensitized stress responses? Or may there be a set of molecular switches that get turned on in key brain cells when people develop addiction, and that underlie, for instance, their stress sensitivity? If these molecular switches indeed do exist, can we find them and hope to reset them? I don't know the answer to this critical question. I suspect that, for now, no one else does either. My dream is of course that those switches do exist and could be switched back. After all, neither would it once have seemed realistic to think it possible to scrape off a skin cell, push three or four molecular buttons, and get it back into a pluripotent embryonic cell stage from which a new individual can be cloned.

If I had to guess, based on what we know today, I would guess that the molecular switches into addiction do exist, as a second, "epigenetic" layer of imprint, a code that determines how the first layer, the genetic code of DNA, is read in different brain cells. We are beginning to see the outlines of that programming. But attempting to target the molecular switches that make up this program code raises some challenging issues. For starters, medications with an ability to turn them on or off may well affect the function of many cells beyond the few brain cells we really want to influence. But it may not necessarily be that way. Not too many years ago, it was thought that these types of medications would never be possible to use in humans, for any indication, because they would have unacceptable toxicity. By now, several of them are in fact used for cancer and seem to be safe and reasonably well tolerated. Never exclude the possibility of unexpected progress.

Meanwhile, one of the most striking aspects of working at the intersection of the science of addiction and the treatment of addictive disorders is the gap between these two worlds. It is easy, based on the science I have shared in this book, to essentially brush aside most of what is currently done with and for people with addictive disorders in the real world of treatment. When I set out to write this book, my ambition was to write a persuasive and provocative argument to that effect. To some extent it is indeed hard to escape that conclusion. If we accept that addictions are medical conditions like any others, do we have a choice but to start applying the standards of evidence-based medicine to their treatment? And yet there may well be more to managing and treating addictions than meets the scientific eye. The stigma of these conditions continues to weigh heavily on the lives of people who experience them, often perhaps just as heavily as the effects of drug use itself. The value of institutions and traditions that safeguard the dignity and humanity of patients with addictive disorders probably neither can nor should be measured only by the scientific standards of medicine. I feel strongly that patients with addictions should have the best treatment science supports, but I am not sure I have the answers to all the difficult questions that arise when traditional treatments and modern science and evidence-based medicine meet.

But I do have at least three overarching questions.

First, can we tolerate that a large proportion of the treatment and recovery community ignores the modern science of addiction and the evidence for new treatments simply because it happens to contradict their interpretation of principles conceived three quarters of a century ago? As we have seen, the disease burden from addiction can now be markedly reduced by treatments that have a solid evidence base. In many cases the failure to provide these treatments means the difference between life and death. In other cases the difference is between a life that can be reasonably productive, healthy, and rich in affection and a life that is burdened by poverty, disease, and progressive social exclusion. In any other area of medicine, failure to provide treatments with known ability to improve outcomes would result in massive lawsuits. When a debate gets started over the rationale for providing expensive cancer treatments that just prolong life by a few months, people start yelling "death panels." Yet when it comes to patients with addictive disorders, no one is held accountable for the failure to provide treatments that provide some of the best documented benefits in clinical medicine.

Part of this question is, of course, about the fact that addiction treatment largely lies outside the world of medicine and health care, which have more or less established standards for what is to be considered reliable evidence. It is easy to be critical of addiction treatment programs that do not apply modern standards of evidence-based medicine. But in doing so, we also need to remember that the medical profession has shown limited interest in claiming this field. In fact, while the science of addiction shows perhaps the greatest advances among complex diseases, and while the progress in science-based treatments is encouraging, addiction medicine continues to have great difficulties in recruiting the numbers and the quality of physicians who could build on these advances and transform the treatment of addictive disorders for large numbers of patients. One of the greatest challenges the field is facing is attracting medical students and young physicians to addiction medicine by showing them the excitement of the science and the opportunities for making a difference clinically. Unless we develop strategies that make us successful in this pursuit, it really does not matter how effective medical treatments that do or do not get developed are. If there is no one to deliver them, they will not be delivered.

Second, if addiction is a chronic, relapsing disorder, then, whatever tools we use based on the evidence, its management has to be the work of a lifetime. Combine that with the insight that most people with addictive disorders largely lack financial resources, and another set of unavoidable questions presents itself. Can a traditional twenty-eight-day residential program, with its cost somewhere in the range of $40,000 and up, continue to be justified under those circumstances, in particular when data show that outpatient-based treatments that apply modern behavioral and pharmacological treatments can achieve equally good or even better outcomes? The emerging emphasis in many of the good programs on continuing care is certainly a move in the right direction. But it does not address this fundamental question. If a given amount of resources is available to treat a patient with an addictive disorder, how are those resources best spent? What amount is it reasonable to spend up-front on an expensive residential treatment, compared with the cost of all the following years of management locally, in the community?

This question is made particularly important as treatment options evolve. How does this balance change as new treatment options for long-term management of addiction emerge? With the emergence of reasonably effective relapse prevention medications for alcoholism such as naltrexone for some patients, or safe and easily managed maintenance treatments for opioid addiction such as buprenorphine, the question of where to devote the most resources becomes critical. As an example, infectious disease medicine closed most of its inpatient wards and transformed itself into largely an outpatient-based specialty as better and better antibiotics arrived on the scene, while science showed that being confined to an expensive hospital bed did not provide much additional benefit. In another case, surgeons who had built careers on developing exquisitely precise nerve-cutting procedures aimed at reducing gastric acid production had to find something else to do once medications such as Tagemet, Zantac, and Losec became available. Surely addiction medicine will have to retool as the science brings forward new approaches?

But this question, too, has a second part. If science shows that the cost of traditional residential treatments cannot be justified in the long term, how do we avoid losing the value that is inherent in established, well-run institutions such as Hazelden? These places have a value beyond the specifics of the treatment they deliver. They also serve as passionate advocates for a patient population that few others care about and are carriers of a culture and tradition that, even absent the beds, have a tremendous value. If nothing is done, then the pressures from insurance companies and other funding sources will leave those institutions with little choice other than scaling down, catering only to a clientele that can pay its own way, or both. That, in turn, would leave the rest of the patient population, who lack those financial resources, without access to institutions committed to restoring their dignity. In the absence of other options, many patients would be back to the situation from which I believe Dan Anderson wanted to create a path out.

Transforming existing treatment programs so that they adapt to the emerging science and practice of evidence-based addiction medicine faces immense challenges. Doing so without losing sight of the guiding principles that were once behind those treatment programs and that to a large extent remain valid brings that challenge to another level. In practical terms, what do you do with 150 beds in a beautiful middle-of-nowhere in Minnesota if you arrive at the conclusion that they are no longer needed? I don't have an answer to that question either. But I do know that unless a good answer is developed, financial realities may drive an answer that patients will not benefit from.

Third, and perhaps most upsetting, how can we get rid of the quacks? Seriously. It is bad enough when people do not receive effective treatments that are available. It is absurd and upsetting when, instead, charlatans are allowed to prey on vulnerable people and get rich from it. I hope to have made a convincing argument that addiction is a disease not much different from other chronic relapsing conditions. I hope to have shown that it is frequently deadly and in other cases results in extensive disability. That being the case, it would be reasonable to expect the same kind of oversight over its treatment as we expect in the case of other serious diseases. Any hospital worker in the United States lives with the knowledge that any day, we may come to work only to meet an inspector from the Joint Commission on Accreditation of Healthcare Organizations. We know that if our practice departs the slightest from science-based standards of care, we will be cited. That will not be done with the objective to punish but rather with the expectation that it will be used as a corrective to improve our practice. Although they are clearly stressful, we basically welcome these inspections and citations. Through them we keep a check on whether we are doing the best we can for our patients. Yet anyone can open shop in Malibu, claim to cure addiction using methods that have no support in the evidence, charge patients made vulnerable by their condition tens of thousands of dollars or more, and get away with it.

While simple and clear-cut in the extreme cases, this question is one that on other occasions also has shades of gray. There is of course a whole spectrum of providers. The bare-bones, publicly funded methadone maintenance program may serve to illustrate one of the extremes. It costs a patient nothing and the community not a whole lot. When done the right way, it provides one of the most effective and cost-effective treatments in clinical medicine, based on decades of good research-quality data. It does not promise a cure but supports a life as free of relapse and its consequences as possible. Places like Passages in Malibu are at the other end of the spectrum, and I have probably made it clear enough how I feel about those. But between these extremes are the Hazeldens, the Betty Ford Clinics, and other programs, with their mixed bag of deference to science, commercialism, and promises of cures. I am reminded that the criticism leveled at these places should not stop there. It is just as bad when physicians offer expensive MR scans of the brain as a standard part of an addiction treatment package, with vague reference to addiction as a brain disease and no science to support any clinical benefit.

I have shared much of what I have learned over the more than twenty years since I started out in this field. Then, I was naïve, enthusiastic, and hopeful. All these years later, I am hopefully somewhat less naïve. Yet I remain as hopeful as ever that science will, in my lifetime, bring forward opportunities for better and better treatments to offer people with addictive disorders. Just in the time I have been in the field, after all quite brief on the timescale of science, progress has been mind-boggling. We have learned so much about brain processes that in some people result in compulsive, self-destructive drug use, depriving them and their loved ones of much of what life has to offer, or life itself.

The behavior of people with addictions is no longer a mystery, at least not entirely. This is certainly true at the behavioral level, at which we know very well what events make people resume drug seeking and drug use. But it is also increasingly true at the level of brain circuits and molecules. Because of advances in the neuroscience of addiction, the list of receptors, enzymes, and other mechanisms we could target with medications to halt, or perhaps even reverse, these processes is already long. My colleagues and I do not need to worry about running out of interesting work before retirement. The possible financial as well as human rewards are immense, fully on the scale of major improvements to treatment of cancer or cardiovascular diseases.

But as I write the final words of this book, I am troubled about whether we as a society will be able to translate current and future scientific breakthroughs in the area of addiction into better lives for patients. Prejudice, stigma, and financial interests conspire to prevent science-based treatments from reaching patients who need them. Will we ever be ready to end treatment of addiction as a business, profitable for some providers yet unhelpful for the large population of patients? That is not a question that can be solved in the lab. That is a question for you.

NOTES

1. US AND THEM

1. http://www.cdc.gov/alcohol/fact-sheets/alcohol-use.htm.
2. P. Anderson et al., "Effectiveness and cost-effectiveness of policies and programmes to reduce the harm caused by alcohol." *Lancet* 373, no. 9682 (2009): 2234–46.

2. A GROCERY STORE THAT CLOSED

1. "Standardized mortality rate," or SMR, is a useful measure of how deadly a drug is. It indicates the risk of dying, within a certain timeframe, for a person who uses the drug compared with a person of the same sex, age, socioeconomic status, etc. who does not use that drug. For heroin-addicted subjects seeking methadone treatment, this measure indicates between twenty- and fiftyfold increased risk of dying.
2. Such data are important for indicating the probability of developing addiction for particular drugs; they are probably less informative when it comes to comparing the addiction liability of different drugs. The social cost of maintaining a nicotine addiction, although increasing, is still in a different league compared with that associated with cocaine addiction.
3. J. Rehm et al., "Global burden of disease and injury and economic cost attributable to alcohol use and alcohol-use disorders." *Lancet* 373, no. 9682 (2009): 2223–33.
4. D. J. Nutt et al., on behalf of Independent Scientific Committee on Drugs, "Drug harms in the UK: A multicriteria decision analysis." *Lancet* 376, no. 9752 (2010): 1558–65. David Nutt was fired as government adviser after reaching these inconvenient conclusions.

5. J. Rehm et al., "The relationship of average volume of alcohol consumption and patterns of drinking to burden of disease: An overview." *Addiction* 98, no. 9 (2003): 1209–28.

6. D. S. Hasin et al., "Prevalence, correlates, disability, and comorbidity of DSM-IV alcohol abuse and dependence in the United States: Results from the National Epidemiologic Survey on Alcohol and Related Conditions." *Archives of General Psychiatry* 64, no. 7 (2007): 830–42.

3. AN ENTITY IN ITS OWN RIGHT

1. I have not been able to establish the species of mushroom in these accounts, but from the description of symptoms, they must have contained substances that block one of the brain receptors for acetylcholin, a transmitter involved in cognition and memory.

2. Much of addiction research has been carried out without appropriate attention to this fact. Although experiments are simpler when animals have access only to the drug studied, that may well create a rather artificial situation. Illustrating this fact, the laboratory of Dr. Serge Ahmed in Bordeaux, France, has elegantly shown that when sugar is available as an alternative, the motivation of rats to obtain cocaine dramatically decreases.

3. J. Anthony et al., "Comparative epidemiology of dependence on tobacco, alcohol, controlled substances, and inhalants: Basic findings from the National Comorbidity Survey." *Experimental and Clinical Psychopharmacology* 2 (1994): 244–68; *National Household Survey on Drug Abuse: Main Findings*, DHHS publication no. (SMA) 00–3381 (Rockville, Md.: Department of Health and Human Services, Substance Abuse and Mental Health Services Administration, 2000). The substances examined included cocaine, other stimulants such as amphetamine, heroin, painkillers, cannabis, tranquilizers, alcohol, and tobacco.

4. A new version is expected in 2017.

5. "Syndrome" comes from Greek, meaning "run together"—a set of features that frequently occur together. It is typically assumed in medicine that a common underlying mechanism causes such features.

6. The American Psychiatric Association, which publishes the *Diagnostic and Statistical Manual of Mental Disorders*, included a category in the fourth edition of the manual (DSM-IV) very similar to the WHO/ICD criteria. The fifth edition (DSM-V), published in October 2013, did away with the abuse/dependence dichotomy, added "craving" as an explicit criterion, and made physical dependence a characteristic of the disorder—say, "alcohol use disorder with/without tolerance/withdrawal."

7. The exceptions are tranquilizers such as Valium and hallucinogens such as LSD.

8. V. Deroche-Gamonet et al., "Evidence for addiction-like behavior in the rat." *Science* 305, no. 5686 (2004): 1014–17; L. J. Vanderschuren and B. J. Everitt, "Drug

seeking becomes compulsive after prolonged cocaine self-administration." *Science* 305, no. 5686 (2004): 1017–19.

9. To quote Alan Leshner, former director of NIDA and one of the most effective communicators I have ever met: "Addiction is a brain disease, and it matters." A. Leshner, "Addiction is a brain disease, and it matters." *Science* 278, no. 5335 (1997): 45–47.

10. That is an American view. Being Jewish, I could claim that what is pursued is decreased misery.

11. Although this may appear dangerously close to circular reasoning, it is not. Depression can be effectively treated in people who also have drug problems. Once treatment gets a handle on both the depression and the substance use, the desire to live is as strong as in anyone else.

12. See, e.g., S. H. Ahmed and G. F. Koob, "Transition from moderate to excessive drug intake: Change in hedonic set point." *Science* 282, no. 5387 (1998): 298–300.

13. H. Kristenson et al., "Identification and intervention of heavy drinking in middle-aged men: Results and follow-up of 24–60 months of long-term study with randomized controls." *Alcoholism: Clinical and Experimental Research* 7, no. 2 (1983): 203–9.

14. D. S. Hasin et al., "Prevalence, correlates, disability, and comorbidity of DSM-IV alcohol abuse and dependence in the United States: Results from the National Epidemiologic Survey on Alcohol and Related Conditions." *Archives of General Psychiatry* 64, no. 7 (2007): 830–42; B. F. Grant et al., "Prevalence and co-occurrence of substance use disorders and independent mood and anxiety disorders: Results from the National Epidemiologic Survey on Alcohol and Related Conditions." *Archives of General Psychiatry* 61, no. 8 (2004): 807–16.

15. R. Culverhouse et al., "Long-term stability of alcohol and other substance dependence diagnoses and habitual smoking: An evaluation after 5 years." *Archives of General Psychiatry* 62, no. 7 (2005): 753–60.

16. A robust cannabinoid withdrawal syndrome can be precipitated by blocking cannabinoid receptors. This withdrawal shares many similarities with that from other addictive drugs but is masked by the slow elimination.

4. A CHRONIC, RELAPSING DISORDER

1. When I took up the job, I discovered that one of the inpatient units prided itself in being a medication-free detox ward. I soon learned this meant that if a patient went into alcohol withdrawal seizures on the unit, the patient would be dragged out into the hall before benzodiazepines were administered to break this potentially life-threatening condition. I had to reassign the nurse manager and threaten to report a few other people to the licensing authorities before this practice stopped.

2. T. McLellan et al., "Drug dependence, a chronic medical illness: Implications for treatment, insurance, and outcomes evaluation." *JAMA* 284, no. 13 (2000): 1689–95.

3. I have one complaint about this paper, and one only. Throughout, it used the term "dependence" for what should have been "addiction." For the sake of consistency, I have used the latter.

4. And, one might add, because half the nurses decided they just don't believe in medications, no matter what the data from controlled trials say.

5. MAN OR MACHINE?

1. The term "deterministic" is used here in a broad sense. Most laws of biology are probabilistic rather than truly and strictly deterministic.

2. D. Premack and G. Woodruff, "Does the chimpanzee have a theory of mind." *Behavioral and Brain Sciences* 1, no. 4 (1978): 515–26.

3. At least after scientists have told the computer to assign fanciful colors to the rather boring numbers generated by statistical algorithms, in turn generated from the even more boring numbers that come off the MR equipment.

4. In Kantian terms, the processes of the brain-mind could be viewed as "the-thing-itself"—*das Ding an sich.*

5. S. Pinker, *The Blank Slate: The Modern Denial of Human Nature* (New York: Penguin, 2002).

6. HISTORIES, BRAINS, AND BEHAVIORS

1. FM stands for "frequency modulated," which is how neurons encode information: a higher-intensity signal is coded by increasing the frequency of impulses, or action potentials, that get sent down the wire (the axon) that takes the signal to the synapse and through the synapse to the next cell.

2. The Nobel Prize in Medicine or Physiology was awarded to Bert Sakmann and Erwin Neher in 1991 for patch clamp electrophysiology, a way of studying electric communication between nerve cells.

3. M. A. Ungless et al., "Single cocaine exposure in vivo induces long-term potentiation in dopamine neurons." *Nature* 411, no. 6837 (2001): 583–87.

4. R. Sinha et al., "Stress-induced cocaine craving and hypothalamic-pituitary-adrenal responses are predictive of cocaine relapse outcomes." *Archives of General Psychiatry* 63, no. 3 (2006): 324–31; R. Sinha et al., "Effects of adrenal sensitivity, stress- and cue-induced craving, and anxiety on subsequent alcohol relapse and treatment outcomes." *Archives of General Psychiatry* 68, no. 9 (2011): 942–52.

5. This statement was made famous in an essay of the same title by the Russian evolutionary biologist Theodosius Dobzhansky in *American Biology Teacher* 35 (1973):

125–29. Although used in the essay to reconcile the author's Christian beliefs with a modern understanding of biology, the statement has much broader implications.

6. D. H. Ingvar, "'Memory of the future': An essay on the temporal organization of conscious awareness." *Human Neurobiology* 4, no. 3 (1985): 127–36.

7. G. F. Koob and N. D. Volkow, "Neurocircuitry of addiction." *Neuropsychopharma-cology* 35, no. 1 (2010): 217–38.

7. THE PURSUIT OF HAPPINESS

1. J. A. Wilson, "Egyptian Secular Songs and Poems," in *Ancient Near Eastern Texts Relating to the Old Testament* (Princeton, N.J.: Princeton University Press, 1969), 467.

2. Note that this operant conditioning is different in a fundamental way from classical, or Pavlovian, conditioning; the latter does not require the subject to exhibit a particular behavior or "operant."

3. This term, a marriage of cognitive psychology and neuroscience, is said to have been coined by George Miller and Michael Gazzaniga in the back seat of a New York taxi. I am happy to provide that observation as experimental support for my hypothesis that being in Manhattan has a powerful influence on the probability of coming up with great ideas.

4. J. Olds and P. Milner, "Positive reinforcement produced by electrical stimulation of septal area and other regions of rat brain." *Journal of Comparative and Physiological Psychology* 47, no. 6 (1954): 419–27; J. Olds, "Self-stimulation of the brain: Its use to study local effects of hunger, sex, and drugs." *Science* 127, no. 3294 (1958): 315–24.

5. J. Olds, in *Brain Stimulation and Reward*, ed. E. S. Valenstein (Glenview, Ill.: Scott, Foresman, 1973).

6. Many hard-core behaviorists to this day do not like to talk about internal states and shrug at the notion that a rat might experience pleasure; thus they use terms such as "hedonic value." Given that the meaning of the Greek root word for "hedonic" is "sweet" and was used to denote things that give pleasure, I find that amusing.

7. V. Deroche-Gamonet et al., "Evidence for addiction-like behavior in the rat." *Science* 305, no. 5686 (2004): 1014–17; L. J. Vanderschuren and B. J. Everitt, "Drug seeking becomes compulsive after prolonged cocaine self-administration." *Science* 305, no. 5686 (2004): 1017–19.

8. R. A. Wise, "Addictive drugs and brain stimulation reward." *Annual Review of Neuroscience* 19 (1996): 319–40.

9. A. Carlsson et al., "3,4-Dihydroxyphenylalanine and 5-hydroxytryptophan as reserpine antagonists." *Nature* 180, no. 4596 (1957): 1200. To understand why Carlsson's discovery was met with such skepticism, one has to realize that the presence of dopamine in the brain was known at the time, but everybody thought they already knew its role there: as an intermediate step along the way to making a "real" neurotransmitter, norephinephrine.

10. Developed by two other Swedes, Bengt Falck and Nils-Åke Hillarp of Lund University, the formaldehyde fluorescence method enabled much of modern neuroscience to get started in the early 1960s. Hillarp was Carlsson's doctoral adviser in Lund. He tragically died from melanoma at the age of forty-nine.

11. The number is much lower, perhaps around twenty-five thousand, in a mouse. It seems that the further we evolve, the more cells the ventral tegmental area contains.

12. The upper part of the basal ganglia, the dorsal striatum, is more directly involved in movement control, and its loss of dopamine input is the disease mechanism of Parkinson's disease.

13. M. A. Bozarth and R. A. Wise, "Toxicity associated with long-term intravenous heroin and cocaine self-administration in the rat." *JAMA* 254, no. 1 (1985): 81–83.

14. T. M. Tzschentke, "Measuring reward with the conditioned place preference (CPP) paradigm: Update of the last decade." *Addiction Biology* 12, no. 3–4 (2007): 227–462.

15. Recently the research group of Harriet de Wit at University of Chicago and work we have done in collaboration with that group have shown that humans will also exhibit conditioned place preference. E. Childs and H. de Wit, "Amphetamine-induced place preference in humans." *Biological Psychiatry* 65, no. 10 (2009): 900–904; L. M. Mayo et al., "Conditioned preference to a methamphetamine-associated contextual cue in humans." *Neuropsychopharmacology* 38 (2013): 921–29.

16. If this all sounds simple, it both is and is not. Conceptually, CPP indeed has an attractive simplicity to it. In practicality, it is extremely sensitive to many irrelevant factors, such as whether one of the two environments is inherently more interesting or more unpleasant for the mouse. CPP is particularly tricky with alcohol, for instance, because higher doses obviously lead to impairment that will get in the way of measuring reward based on how the mouse moves around.

17. R. A. Wise and M. A. Bozarth, "A psychomotor stimulant theory of addiction." *Psychology Review* 94, no. 4 (1987): 469–92.

18. G. Di Chiara and A. Imperato, "Drugs abused by humans preferentially increase synaptic dopamine concentrations in the mesolimbic system of freely moving rats." *Proceedings of the National Academy of Science USA* 85, no. 14 (1988): 5274–78.

19. E.g., N. Volkow et al., "Relationship between subjective effects of cocaine and dopamine transporter occupancy." *Nature* 386, no. 6627 (1997): 827–30; N. Volkow et al., "Reinforcing effects of psychostimulants in humans are associated with increases in brain dopamine and occupancy of D(2) receptors." *Journal of Pharmacology and Experimental Therapeutics* 291, no. 1 (1999): 409–15.

20. W. Schultz, "Predictive reward signal of dopamine neurons." *Journal of Neurophysiology* 80 (1998): 1–27.

21. S. E. Hyman et al., "Neural mechanisms of addiction: The role of reward-related learning and memory." *Annual Review of Neuroscience* 29 (2006): 565–98.

22. A. Badiani et al., "Opiate versus psychostimulant addiction: The differences do matter." *Nature Reviews Neuroscience* 12, no. 11 (2011): 685–700.

23. K. Kiianmaa et al., "On the role of ascending dopamine systems in the control of voluntary ethanol intake and ethanol intoxication." *Pharmacology Biochemistry and Behavior* 10, no. 4 (1979): 603–8; Z. Amit and Z. W. Brown, "Actions of drugs of abuse on brain reward systems: A reconsideration with specific attention to alcohol." *Pharmacology Biochemistry and Behavior* 17, no. 2 (1982): 233–38; S. Rassnick et al., "The effects of 6-hydroxydopamine lesions of the nucleus accumbens and the mesolimbic dopamine system on oral self-administration of ethanol in the rat." *Brain Research* 623, no. 1 (1993): 16–24.

24. I. Boileau et al., "Alcohol promotes dopamine release in the human nucleus accumbens." *Synapse* 49, no. 4 (2003): 226–31; J. M. Gilman et al., "Why we like to drink: A functional magnetic resonance imaging study of the rewarding and anxiolytic effects of alcohol." *Journal of Neuroscience* 28, no. 18 (2008): 4583–91.

25. N. B. Urban et al., "Sex differences in striatal dopamine release in young adults after oral alcohol challenge: A positron emission tomography imaging study with [^{11}C]raclopride." *Biological Psychiatry* 68, no. 8 (2010): 689–96.

26. V. A. Ramchandani et al., "A genetic determinant of the striatal dopamine response to alcohol in men." *Molecular Psychiatry* 16, no. 8 (2011): 809–17.

27. J. M. Gilman et al., "Subjective and neural responses to intravenous alcohol in young adults with light and heavy drinking patterns." *Neuropsychopharmacology* 37, no. 2 (2012): 467–77.

28. T. Robinson and K. Berridge, "Addiction." *Annual Review of Psychology* 54 (2003): 25–53.

29. K. Berridge et al., "Dissecting components of reward: 'Liking,' 'wanting,' and learning." *Current Opinion in Pharmacology* 9 (2009): 65–73.

30. A. J. Machin and R. I. M. Dunbar, "The brain opioid theory of social attachment: A review of the evidence." *Behaviour* 148 (2011): 985–1025.

31. C. Pert and S. Snyder, "Opiate receptor: Demonstration in nervous tissue." *Science* 179, no. 4077 (1973): 1011–14.

32. L. Terenius and A. Wahlstrom, "Search for an endogenous ligand for the opiate receptor." *Acta Physiologica Scandinavica* 94, no. 1 (1975): 74–81.

33. J. Hughes et al., "Identification of two related pentapeptides from the brain with potent opiate agonist activity." *Nature* 258, no. 5536 (1975): 577–80.

34. R. Kanigel, *Apprentice to Genius: The Making of a Scientific Dynasty* (Baltimore: Johns Hopkins University Press, 1993).

35. Mu-opioid receptors are of course plentiful in numerous other brain areas and are involved in many other brain functions. The ones listed are simply a selection of those most relevant for our discussion.

36. A. M. Graybiel, "Habits, rituals, and the evaluative brain." *Annual Review of Neuroscience* 31 (2008): 359–87.

37. A. L. Milton and B. J. Everitt, "The persistence of maladaptive memory: Addiction, drug memories and anti-relapse treatments." *Neuroscience and Biobehavioral Reviews* 36, no. 4 (2012): 1119–39.

38. Robinson and Berridge, "Addiction."
39. D. Morgan et al., "Social dominance in monkeys: Dopamine D2 receptors and cocaine self-administration." *Nature Neuroscience* 5, no. 2 (2002): 169–74.
40. N. D. Volkow et al., "Prediction of reinforcing responses to psychostimulants in humans by brain dopamine D2 receptor levels." *American Journal of Psychiatry* 156, no. 9 (1999): 1440–43.

8. THE DARK SIDE OF ADDICTION

1. Proverbs 31:6.
2. E. J. Khantzian et al., "Heroin use as an attempt to cope: clinical observations." *American Journal of Psychiatry* 131, no. 2 (1974): 160–64; Khantzian, "The self-medication hypothesis of substance use disorders: A reconsideration and recent applications." *Harvard Review of Psychiatry* 4, no. 5 (1997): 231–44.
3. D. F. Duncan, "Reinforcement of drug abuse: Implications for prevention." *Clinical Toxicology Bulletin* 4, no. 2 (1974): 69–75.
4. D. A. Regier et al., "Comorbidity of mental disorders with alcohol and other drug abuse: Results from the Epidemiologic Catchment Area (ECA) Study." *JAMA* 264, no. 19 (1990): 2511–18.
5. C. A. Dackis and M. S. Gold, "More on self-medication and drug abuse." *American Journal of Psychiatry* 143, no. 10 (1986): 1309–10; M. A. Schuckit and V. Hesselbrock, "Alcohol dependence and anxiety disorders: What is the relationship?" *American Journal of Psychiatry* 151, no. 12 (1994): 1723–34; R. J. Frances, "The wrath of grapes versus the self-medication hypothesis." *Harvard Review of Psychiatry* 4, no. 5 (1997): 287–89.
6. G. F. Koob and F. E. Bloom, "Cellular and molecular mechanisms of drug dependence." *Science* 242, no. 4879 (1988): 715–23.
7. R. L. Solomon and J. D. Corbit, "An opponent-process theory of motivation. I. Temporal dynamics of affect." *Psychology Review* 81, no. 2 (1974): 119–45.
8. P. Sterling and J. Eyer, "Allostasis: A New Paradigm to Explain Arousal Pathology." In *Handbook of Life Stress, Cognition and Health*, ed. S. Fisher and J. Reason (New York: Wiley, 1988).
9. B. S. McEwen, *The End of Stress as We Know It* (Washington, D.C.: Joseph Henry Press, 2004).
10. D. B. Goldstein and N. Pal, "Alcohol dependence produced in mice by inhalation of ethanol: Grading the withdrawal reaction." *Science* 172, no. 3980 (1971): 288–90.
11. M. Heilig and G. F. Koob, "A key role for corticotropin-releasing factor in alcohol dependence." *Trends in Neurosciences* 30, no. 8 (2007): 399–406.
12. S. H. Ahmed and G. F. Koob, "Transition from moderate to excessive drug intake: Change in hedonic set point." *Science* 282, no. 5387 (1998): 298–300; S. H. Ahmed et al., "Neurobiological evidence for hedonic allostasis associated with escalating cocaine use." *Nature Neuroscience* 5, no. 7 (2002): 625–26.

9. RASH ACTIONS

1. Economic decision-making theory frequently refers to "utility" as an intrinsic metric of a reward; in contrast, "subjective value" is that utility, discounted by the individual for various factors such as, e.g., how long into the future the reward lies, how uncertain it may be, etc.

2. I use "light up" here in a loose sense that refers to increased activity. Most of the time we would apply different methods to follow the brain activity in the rat and the human, although advances in imaging technology actually now make it possible to apply some methods much the same way in both cases.

3. For a great review of the somatic marker theory, see A. Bechara et al., "Emotion, decision making and the orbitofrontal cortex." *Cerebral Cortex* 10, no. 3 (2000): 295–307. Damasio has also published a fascinating popular account of this uniquely human functionality in his book *Descartes' Error: Emotion, Reason, and the Human Brain* (New York: Putnam, 1994).

4. K. R. Ridderinkhof et al., "The role of the medial frontal cortex in cognitive control." *Science* 306, no. 5695 (2004): 443–47.

5. Or are at least key players in those functions; in reality, no brain structure does anything entirely on its own.

6. This seemingly simple function of the brain, how many things we can hold in memory at a given time, is in fact so important that it seems to influence academic achievement more than the global IQ measure. T. P. Alloway and R. G. Alloway, "Investigating the predictive roles of working memory and IQ in academic attainment." *Journal of Experimental Child Psychology* 106, no. 1 (2010): 20–29.

7. Reviewed in W. Mischel et al., "Delay of gratification in children." *Science* 244, no. 4907 (1989): 933–28.

8. A once popular hypothesis of development held that "ontogenesis recapitulates phylogenesis," meaning that the development of the embryo follows that of the species. Although not uniformly true for all embryonic development, it is generally the rule that cognitive achievements that are the most recent in the evolutionary history of a species are also the ones to come online last during development of the individual.

9. U.S. Supreme Court, *Graham* v. *Florida*, 2010.

10. B. J. Casey et al., "Behavioral and neural correlates of delay of gratification 40 years later." *Proceedings of the National Academy of Science USA* 108, no. 36 (2011): 14998–15003.

11. H. de Wit, "Impulsivity as a determinant and consequence of drug use: A review of underlying processes." *Addiction Biology* 14, no. 1 (2009): 22–31.

12. T. E. Wilens et al., "Does stimulant therapy of attention-deficit/hyperactivity disorder beget later substance abuse? A meta-analytic review of the literature." *Pediatrics* 111, no. 1 (2003): 179–85..

13. T. Klingberg et al., "Computerized training of working memory in children with ADHD—a randomized, controlled trial." *Journal of the American Academy of Child and Adolescent Psychiatry* 44, no. 2 (2005): 177–86.

NOTES

14. J. D. Jentsch and J. R. Taylor, "Impulsivity resulting from frontostriatal dysfunction in drug abuse: Implications for the control of behavior by reward-related stimuli." *Psychopharmacology* (Berlin) 146, no. 4 (1999): 373–90; de Wit, "Impulsivity as a determinant and consequence of drug use"; J. M. Gilman et al., "The effect of intravenous alcohol on the neural correlates of risky decision making in healthy social drinkers." *Addiction Biology* 17, no. 2 (2012): 465–78.

15. P. T. Mehlman et al., "Low CSF 5-HIAA concentrations and severe aggression and impaired impulse control in nonhuman primates." *American Journal of Psychiatry* 151, no. 10 (1994): 1485–91; D. Higley and M. Linnoila, "A nonhuman primate model of excessive alcohol intake: Personality and neurobiological parallels of type I- and type II-like alcoholism." *Recent Developments in Alcoholism* 13 (1997): 191–219.

16. D. Belin et al., "High impulsivity predicts the switch to compulsive cocaine-taking." *Science* 320, no. 5881 (2008): 1352–55.

17. A. Damasio et al., "The return of Phineas Gage: Clues about the brain from the skull of a famous patient." *Science* 264, no. 5162 (1994): 1102–5.

18. http://www.slate.com/articles/health_and_science/science/2014/05/ phineas_gage _neuroscience_case_true_story_of_famous_frontal_lobe_patient.html.

10. TURNING ON A BRIGHT LIGHT

1. I work obsessively with patients to reconstruct the chain of events leading up to a relapse in petty detail, which invariably requires revisiting the issue several times. It is amazing how often the initial answer to the simple question, "What happened?" is "I have no idea—all of a sudden I was drinking," only to ultimately emerge as a logical process that the patient looks at and says, "How could I fool myself like that?" As we will see in a later chapter, behavioral analysis of that kind is a key element of relapse prevention treatment.

2. Harriet subsequently came to establish a highly successful research group at University of Chicago and remains to date at the forefront of human psychopharmacology and addiction research.

3. Y. Shaham et al., "The reinstatement model of drug relapse: History, methodology and major findings." *Psychopharmacology* (Berlin) 168, nos. 1–2 (2003): 3–20; D. H. Epstein et al., "Toward a model of drug relapse: An assessment of the validity of the reinstatement procedure." *Psychopharmacology* (Berlin) 189, no. 1 (2006):1–16.

4. Work by Anh Dzung Lê and colleagues at the University of Toronto suggests that in the case of alcohol, priming is less potent than other stimuli, such as stress, in triggering relapse in rats. This is not the case with other drugs when these are studied in rats or in patients. I don't know why this is. After all, it is not too shocking that there are limits to similarities between drug-seeking behavior in rats and humans.

5. This has been studied most extensively for reinstatement of cocaine seeking and to

274

some extent that of heroin seeking, pointing to neighboring but somewhat different parts of the frontal lobes.

6. This insight parallels critical studies on extinction of learned fear by Joseph LeDoux
in the 1990s.

7. J. R. Volpicelli et al., "Naltrexone in the treatment of alcohol dependence." *Archives
of General Psychiatry* 49, no. 11 (1992): 876–80.

8. American as well as European studies, by Linda Sobell and Mats Berglund, respectively, have suggested that some individuals with established alcoholism may in fact
be able to successfully return to controlled drinking. But these are a minority, there
is no way of knowing who they are ahead of time, and the consequences of relapse
to heavy drinking can be disastrous for those who find they do not belong to that
group. So my advice stands. Given the stakes, it seems reasonable to err on the side
of caution.

11. GETTING THE CUE

1. C. P. O'Brien et al., "Conditioned narcotic withdrawal in humans." *Science* 195, no.
4282 (1977): 1000–1002. The drug was naloxone, an injectable cousin of naltrexone,
both of which I will discuss later. Both these drugs effectively block the mu-opioid
receptor through which heroin produces its addictive effects. Subjects were maintained on methadone, and so the administration of naloxone in an instant reproduced a situation in which the addict is coming off heroin.

2. Although to a lesser degree, opiate addiction remains an occupational hazard
among physicians with easy access to these medications

3. A. Wikler, "Dynamics of drug dependence: Implications of a conditioning theory
for research and treatment." *Archives of General Psychiatry* 28, no. 5 (1973): 611–16.

4. The baso-lateral amygdala, or BLA for short.

5. For a hilarious and thought-provoking review of this topic, see one of the classics
of modern psychology: R. E. Nisbett and T. D. Wilson, "Telling more than we can
know—verbal reports on mental processes." *Psychology Review* 84, no. 3 (1977): 231–59.

6. S. Grant et al., "Activation of memory circuits during cue-elicited cocaine craving."
Proceedings of the National Academy of Science USA 93, no. 21 (1996): 12040–45.

7. A PET scan does not have the resolution to reliably distinguish between different
parts of this structure, so we don't know if these are *exactly* the same regions as
those identified in the animal studies. But they are close enough.

8. H. Myrick et al., "Differential brain activity in alcoholics and social drinkers to
alcohol cues: Relationship to craving." *Neuropsychopharmacology* 29, no. 2 (2004):
393–402.

9. P. W. Kalivas and N. D. Volkow, "The neural basis of addiction: A pathology of
motivation and choice." *American Journal of Psychiatry* 162, no. 8 (2005): 1403–13.

10. R. K. Hester and W. R. Miller, *Handbook of Alcoholism Treatment Approaches: Effective Alternatives* (Boston: Allyn and Bacon, 2003).

11. Over decades of work, LeDoux has made some of the most important discoveries in the understanding of the biology of emotions. He has also written the best introductory text on the topic, the informative and enjoyable *The Emotional Brain: The Mysterious Underpinnings of Emotional Life* (New York: Simon and Schuster, 1996). Although targeting an educated lay audience, that text is required reading for all new students and postdocs in my lab.

12. K. Nader et al., "Fear memories require protein synthesis in the amygdala for reconsolidation after retrieval." *Nature* 406, no. 6797 (2000): 722–26; M. H. Monfils et al., "Extinction-reconsolidation boundaries: key to persistent attenuation of fear memories." *Science* 324, no. 5929 (2009): 951–55.

13. Y. X. Xue et al., "A memory retrieval-extinction procedure to prevent drug craving and relapse." *Science* 336, no. 6078 (2012): 241–45.

12. A STRAINED MIND

1. The names, places, and details of this account have been altered to de-identify them. The salient facts of the experience have not.

2. R. Sinha et al., "Effects of adrenal sensitivity, stress- and cue-induced craving, and anxiety on subsequent alcohol relapse and treatment outcomes." *Archives of General Psychiatry* 68, no. 9 (2011): 942–52; R. Sinha et al., "Stress-induced cocaine craving and hypothalamic-pituitary-adrenal responses are predictive of cocaine relapse outcomes." *Archives of General Psychiatry* 63, no. 3 (2006): 324–31.

3. A small, initial treatment trial would typically require 150–200 subjects, each of them treated for three to six months, and cost around $10 million.

4. According to medical convention, a "factor" is a hypothetical entity that has not yet been identified. Once it is purified and its molecular nature determined, it is elevated to a real "hormone." CRF's discoverer Wylie Vale stuck with the label "factor." Out of respect for his great discovery, so did many of his trainees and collaborators. As a result, both names are now used, with medical textbooks often using the term "hormone," that is, CRH.

5. Cortisol is the main stress hormone in humans and nonhuman primates. Its chemical relative corticosterone functions in this role in commonly used laboratory animals such as rats or mice. To avoid constantly making this distinction, researchers frequently use the abbreviation "cort," which can refer to either of these.

6. For an in-depth explanation of stress physiology combined with hilarious fun, see R. Sapolsky, *Why Zebras Don't Get Ulcers* (New York: Holt, 2004). Science for nonscientists doesn't get better than that.

7. W. Vale et al., "Characterization of a 41-residue ovine hypothalamic peptide that stimulates secretion of corticotropin and beta-endorphin." *Science* 213, no. 4514 (1981): 1394–97.

8. N. Eisenberger et al., "Does rejection hurt? An FMRI study of social exclusion." *Science* 302, no. 5643 (2003): 290–92.

9. N. H. Naqvi et al., "Damage to the insula disrupts addiction to cigarette smoking." *Science* 315, no. 5811 (2007): 531–34.

10. P. Maurage et al., "Disrupted regulation of social exclusion in alcohol-dependence: An FMRI study." *Neuropsychopharmacology* 37, no. 9 (2012): 2067–75.

13. FATHERS AND SONS

1. This particular saying may be equally or even more important in reminding us of the role of fetal alcohol exposure in reprogramming the brain.

2. R. C. Lewontin et al., *Not in Our Genes: Biology, Ideology, and Human Nature* (New York: Pantheon, 1985).

3. J. Locke, "An essay concerning human understanding" (1890). Although famous for this concept in modern times, Locke is not its originator. In the first psychology textbook ever written, *De Anima*, Aristotle wrote about the mind literally as "an unscribed tablet." It seems, however, that this proposition did not gain much traction for a millennium or so.

4. In his highly recommended book *The Blank Slate: The Modern Denial of Human Nature* (New York: Penguin, 2002), Steven Pinker traces the origins of this notion, analyzes its influence in many areas of modern thought, and picks it apart in ways that are brilliant, funny, and ultimately necessary.

5. C. R. Cloninger et al., "Inheritance of alcohol abuse: Cross-fostering analysis of adopted men." *Archives of General Psychiatry* 38, no. 8 (1981): 861–68. The temperance boards have long disappeared.

6. D. W. Goodwin et al., "Drinking problems in adopted and nonadopted sons of alcoholics." *Archives of General Psychiatry* 31, no. 2 (1974): 164–69.

7. S. Sigvardsson et al., "Replication of the Stockholm Adoption Study of alcoholism: Confirmatory cross-fostering analysis." *Archives of General Psychiatry* 53, no. 8 (1981): 681–87.

8. This is called "the equal environment assumption" (EEA) and was for a while under some debate. Although a legitimate methodological concern, it was frequently invoked as a last-ditch effort to dismiss robust findings of a genetic risk in behavioral disorders. This was largely put to rest by Ken Kendler of Virginia Commonwealth University, using real-world data—see e.g. Kendler et al., "Parental treatment and the equal environment assumption in twin studies of psychiatric illness." *Psychological Medicine* 24, no. 3 (1994): 579–90.

9. D. Goldman et al., "The genetics of addictions: uncovering the genes." *Nature Reviews Genetics* 6, no. 7 (2005): 521–32.

10. T. J. Bouchard and M. McGue, "Genetic and environmental influences on human psychological differences." *Journal of Neurobiology* 54, no. 1 (2003): 4–45.

11. E. Turkheimer et al., "Socioeconomic status modifies heritability of IQ in young children." *Psychological Science* 14, no. 6 (2003): 623–28.

12. M. Heilig et al., "Pharmacogenetic approaches to the treatment of alcohol addiction." *Nature Reviews Neuroscience* 12, no. 11 (2011): 670–84.

13. K. S. Kendler et al., "The structure of genetic and environmental risk factors for common psychiatric and substance use disorders in men and women." *Archives of General Psychiatry* 60, no. 9 (2003): 929–37.

14. Schuckit was first a medical student and then a resident at Washington University, an environment shaped by several pioneers of early psychiatric genetics. He frequently speaks of the formative influence and inspiration of that environment. Great places like that are what helps great people grow.

15. M. A. Schuckit, "Low level of response to alcohol as a predictor of future alcoholism." *American Journal of Psychiatry* 151, no. 2 (1994): 184–89; M. A. Schuckit, T. L. Smith, "An 8-year follow-up of 450 sons of alcoholic and control subjects." *Archives of General Psychiatry* 53, no. 3 (1996): 202.

16. M. B. Stein and D. J. Stein, "Social anxiety disorder." *Lancet* 371, no. 9618 (2008): 1115–25.

17. Danielle studies impulsivity and has applied this concept just to that specific domain of behavioral traits, which itself needs to be "deconstructed" into its components. But the idea applies more broadly to addiction as a concept.

18. I. I. Gottesman and T. D. Gould, "The endophenotype concept in psychiatry: Etymology and strategic intentions." *American Journal of Psychiatry* 160, no. 4 (2003): 636–45.

19. See, e.g., *New York Times*, April 18, 1991.

20. Other examples of genetic variation are chromosome rearrangements, where pieces of a chromosome get broken off from their right place and attached somewhere else, such as in some leukemias, or where a whole chromosome is duplicated, such as in Down syndrome. These types of variation are less common and typically result in much more severe consequences.

21. H. J. Edenberg et al., "Variations in GABRA2, encoding the alpha 2 subunit of the GABA(A) receptor, are associated with alcohol dependence and with brain oscillations." *American Journal of Human Genetics* 74, no. 4 (2004): 705–14.

22. T. E. Thorgeirsson et al., "A variant associated with nicotine dependence, lung cancer and peripheral arterial disease." *Nature* 452, no. 7187 (2008): 638–42.

23. L. E. Hong et al., "A genetically modulated, intrinsic cingulate circuit supports human nicotine addiction." *Proceedings of the National Academy of Science USA* 107, no. 30 (2010): 13509–14.

24. L. Bevilacqua et al., "A population-specific HTR2B stop codon predisposes to severe impulsivity." *Nature* 468, no. 7327 (2010): 1061–66.

14. MOLECULAR CULPRITS

1. See, e.g., R. L. Miller, *The Encyclopedia of Addictive Drugs* (Westport, Conn.: Greenwood Press, 2002).
2. J. O. Josefsson and P. Johansson, "Naloxone-reversible effect of opioids on pinocytosis in Amoeba proteus." *Nature* 282, no. 5734 (1979): 78–80.
3. So named by the Swedish botanist Carl Linnaeus.
4. Since the name of the plant from which the drug is extracted, *Papaver somniferum*, means the "sleep-giving poppy," the new substance is named after the Greek god of sleep and dreams, Morpheus.
5. A British chemist, Charles Romley Wright, had been the first to synthesize heroin, in 1874, but does not seem to have pursued his discovery further.
6. The recovery may take longer after use of very long-lasting opioids, such as methadone.
7. The exceptions are when people in the absence of treatment lose so much fluid that they need an intravenous line to replace it, but that is still not a big deal.
8. E. L. C. Merrall et al., "Meta-analysis of drug-related deaths soon after release from prison." *Addiction* 105, no. 9 (2010): 1545–54.
9. E. Poeppig, *Reise in Peru, Chile und auf dem Amazonenstrohme während der Jahre 1827–32*, reviewed in English in *Journal of the Geographical Society of London* 6 (1836): 381–85.
10. J. V. Lloyd, "Coca, divine plant of the Incas," *Bulletin of Lloyd Library, Cincinnati, Ohio*, pharrn. ser. 4, bull. 18 (1911): 18–25.
11. P. Mantegazza, "On the hygienic and medicinal properties of coca and on nervine nourishment in general," Milan, 1858.
12. H. Markel, *An Anatomy of Addiction: Sigmund Freud, William Halsted and the Miracle Drug, Cocaine* (New York: Pantheon, 2011).
13. B. Giros et al., "Hyperlocomotion and indifference to cocaine and amphetamine in mice lacking the dopamine transporter." *Nature* 379, no. 6566 (379): 606–12.
14. Most people think that this is what the word "paranoia" means. It isn't. Paranoia (from Greek *para*: "outside," and *nous*: "intellect") literally means "delusion" in Greek. "Paranoid delusions" would be to say "delusional delusions."
15. The effects of alcohol on GABA signals is in some ways similar to those produced by the group of antianxiety drugs called benzodiazepines, of which Valium and Librium are probably the most famous members. This explains the many similarities between alcohol and benzodiazepine actions, and also why people addicted to either of those can substitute them for each other.

15. TRICK OR TREATMENT

1. The wording is taken from the Web version of the same ad.
2. Clinical research distinguishes between "effectiveness," which is what we ultimately really want, and "efficacy," which is what we can establish in a reasonable clinical trial. The former is an ability to improve a meaningful clinical outcome—say, reduce mortality from stroke—when treatment is given to regular patients under real-world conditions. The latter is an ability to improve some potentially beneficial clinical measure—say, lower blood pressure—in the people included in a clinical trial, under the rather artificial conditions of that trial.
3. J. Lind, *A Treatise of the Scurvy* (Edinburgh: Sands, Murray, and Cochran, 1753).
4. The NIH, often viewed as a monolith, is in fact a group of disease-oriented institutes, in this case the National Institute on Alcohol Abuse and Alcoholism and the National Institute on Drug Abuse.
5. A better but somewhat less intuitive measure is Cohen's D. Having one of these measures and knowing a couple of other things, one can calculate the other, but the math is not obvious and would take us too far.
6. There is, of course, a whole nonmedical industry that does just that, perhaps not with cancer but certainly with hypertension, diabetes, and other fundamentally medical conditions. This industry, why you should not fall prey to it, and the history and foundations of evidence-based medicine are described in entertaining and informative ways in E. Ernst and S. Singh, *Trick or Treatment: The Undeniable Facts About Alternative Medicine* (New York: Norton, 2008).
7. R. K. Hester and W. R. Miller, *Handbook of Alcoholism Treatment Approaches: Effective Alternatives* (Boston: Allyn and Bacon, 1989).
8. See, e.g., A. T. McLellan et al., "The addiction severity index at 25: Origins, contributions, and transitions." *American Journal of Addiction* 15, no. 2 (2006): 113–24.
9. A. Bandura, "Self-efficacy—toward a unifying theory of behavioral change." *Psychology Review* 84, no. 2 (1977): 191–215.

16. PLEASE BEHAVE

1. B. L. Burke, "The efficacy of motivational interviewing: A meta-analysis of controlled clinical trials." *Journal of Consulting and Clinical Psychology* 71, no. 5 (2003): 843–61.
2. J. B. Saunders et al., "Development of the Alcohol Use Disorders Identification Test (AUDIT): WHO Collaborative Project on Early Detection of Persons with Harmful Alcohol Consumption—II." *Addiction* 88, no. 6 (1993): 791–804; available from the NIAAA at http://pubs.niaaa.nih.gov/publications/Practitioner/Clinicians Guide2005/clinicians_guide11.htm.

NOTES

3. A. Moyer et al., "Brief interventions for alcohol problems: A meta-analytic review of controlled investigations in treatment-seeking and non-treatment-seeking populations." *Addiction* 97, no. 3 (2002): 279–92.
4. M. Berglund et al., *Treating Alcohol and Drug Abuse: An Evidence Based Review* (Weinheim: Wiley-VCH, 2003).
5. E. V. Nunes and F. R. Levin, "Treatment of depression in patients with alcohol or other drug dependence: A meta-analysis." *JAMA* 291, no. 15 (2004): 1887–96.
6. I really don't like this term. There are no "toxins" from which the body needs to be cleansed to initiate abstinence. But the proper alternative is "medically assisted withdrawal," which is just too long.
7. T. H. Brandon et al., "Relapse and relapse prevention." *Annual Review of Clinical Psychology* 3 (2007): 257–84.
8. E. L. C. Merrall et al., "Meta-analysis of drug-related deaths soon after release from prison." *Addiction* 105, no. 9 (2010): 1545–54.
9. K. Witkiewitz and G. A. Marlatt, "Relapse prevention for alcohol and drug problems: That was Zen, this is Tao." *American Psychologist* 59, no. 4 (2004): 224–35.
10. Actually, it is all behavioral. Cognitions are behaviors, too. There is no difference, in principle, between sending electric impulses to muscles to initiate movement and sending them to neurons to initiate thoughts. But that is a separate discussion.
11. D. Epstein et al., "Real-time electronic diary reports of cue exposure and mood in the hours before cocaine and heroin craving and use." *Archives of General Psychiatry* 66, no. 1 (2009): 88–94.
12. J. Peters et al., "Extinction circuits for fear and addiction overlap in prefrontal cortex." *Learning and Memory* 16, no. 5 (2009): 279–88.
13. P. Monti, *Treating Alcohol Dependence: A Coping Skills Training Guide*. 2nd ed. (New York: Guilford Press, 2002).
14. M. Prendergast et al., "Contingency management for treatment of substance use disorders: A meta-analysis." *Addiction* 101, no. 11 (2006): 1546–60.
15. V. Hunot et al., "'Third wave' cognitive and behavioural therapies versus other psychological therapies for depression." *Cochrane Database of Systematic Reviews 2013*, issue 10, art. no. CD008704. DOI: 10.1002/14651858.CD008704.

17. PILLS FOR ADDICTION ILLS

1. The more standard nomenclature, which I have followed, is "opioid receptors," that is, receptors for substances that are either opiates themselves, such as, prototypically, morphine, or similar to those, and so in Greek -*oid* (as in "android," "like a human").
2. R. P. Mattick et al., "Methadone maintenance therapy versus no opioid replacement therapy for opioid dependence." *Cochrane Database of Systematic Reviews* 2009, no. 3: CD002209.

3. A. T. McLellan et al., "The effects of psychosocial services in substance abuse treatment." *JAMA* 269, no. 15 (1993): 1953–59.

4. K. L. Sees et al., "Methadone maintenance vs 180-day psychosocially enriched detoxification for treatment of opioid dependence: A randomized controlled trial." *JAMA* 283, no. 10 (2000): 1303–10.

5. See, e.g., L. M. Gunne et al., "Treatment characteristics and retention in methadone maintenance: High and stable retention rates in a Swedish two-phase programme." *Heroin Addiction and Related Clinical Problems* 4, no. 1 (2002): 37.

6. J. Kakko et al., "A stepped care strategy using buprenorphine and methadone versus conventional methadone maintenance in heroin dependence: A randomized controlled trial." *American Journal of Psychiatry* 164, no. 5 (2007): 797–803.

7. L. Gronbladh et al., "Mortality in heroin addiction: Impact of methadone treatment." *Acta Psychiatrica Scandinavica* 82, no. 3 (1990): 223–27.

8. National Institute on Drug Abuse, Johns Hopkins University, and Reckitt Benckiser. Many people deserve credit, but the one I cannot leave out is Ed Johnson, the pharmacist who made much of this happen both while at Hopkins and after he transitioned to the industry.

9. R. E. Johnson et al., "A comparison of levomethadyl acetate, buprenorphine, and methadone for opioid dependence." *New England Journal of Medicine* 343, no. 18 (2003): 1290–97.

10. R. P. Mattick et al., "Buprenorphine maintenance versus placebo or methadone maintenance for opioid dependence." *Cochrane Database of Systematic Reviews* 2008, no. 2: CD002207.

11. J. Kakko et al., "1-year retention and social function after buprenorphine-assisted relapse prevention treatment for heroin dependence in Sweden: A randomised, placebo-controlled trial." *Lancet* 361, no. 9358 (361): 662–68.

12. D. A. Fiellin et al., "Counseling plus buprenorphine-naloxone maintenance therapy for opioid dependence." *New England Journal of Medicine* 355, no. 4 (2006): 365–74.

13. When taken by the mouth, naloxone will not reach the brain or other interior organs. But it will still be present in the gut, which in a way is on the "outside" of the body. The constipation I described that methadone patients experience and that is also a problem when cancer pain is treated with opioid painkillers turns out to be an effect of opioid receptor activation in the gut. When naloxone is taken by mouth, for example, as an additive to the methadone syrup, the gut receptors will still be blocked, and constipation will be less of a problem. Quite a useful application of pharmacology.

14. P. J. Fudala et al., "Office-based treatment of opiate addiction with a sublingual-tablet formulation of buprenorphine and naloxone." *New England Journal of Medicine* 349, no. 10 (2003): 949–58.

15. These days I don't even have to think about it—as a U.S. government employee, I am simply not allowed to have one.

16. S. Minozzi et al., "Oral naltrexone maintenance treatment for opioid dependence." *Cochrane Database of Systematic Reviews* 2011, no. 4: CD001333.

17. S. D. Comer et al., "Injectable, sustained-release naltrexone for the treatment of opioid dependence: A randomized, placebo-controlled trial." *Archives of General Psychiatry* 63, no. 2 (2006): 210–18.

18. Kakko et al., "A stepped care strategy using buprenorphine and methadone versus conventional methadone maintenance in heroin dependence."

19. L. F. Stead et al., "Nicotine replacement therapy for smoking cessation." *Cochrane Database of Systematic Reviews* 2008, no. 1: CD000146.

20. K. Cahill et al., "Nicotine receptor partial agonists for smoking cessation." *Cochrane database of systematic reviews* 2012, no. 4: CD006103.

21. There are different types of nicotinic receptors. One important category sends signals from nerves to muscles. These are only blocked to put people down for surgery and if blocked otherwise would make smokers quit more than their smoking.

22. R. Spanagel, "Alcoholism: A systems approach from molecular physiology to addictive behavior." *Physiological Reviews* 89, no. 2 (2009): 649–705.

23. M. Heilig et al., "Pharmacogenetic approaches to the treatment of alcohol addiction." *Nature Reviews Neuroscience*12, no. 11 (2011): 670–84.

24. C. H. Jorgensen et al., "The efficacy of disulfiram for the treatment of alcohol use disorder." *Alcoholism: Clinical and Experimental Research* 35, no. 10 (2011): 1749–58.

25. H. L. Altshuler et al., "Alteration of ethanol self-administration by naltrexone." *Life Sciences* 26, no. 9 (1980): 679–88.

26. J. Volpicelli et al., "Naltrexone in the treatment of alcohol dependence." *Archives of General Psychiatry* 49, no. 11 (1992): 876–80; S. O'Malley et al., "Naltrexone and coping skills therapy for alcohol dependence: A controlled study." *Archives of General Psychiatry* 49, no. 11 (1992): 881–87.

27. S. Rosner et al., "Opioid antagonists for alcohol dependence." *Cochrane Database of Systematic Reviews* 2010, no. 12: CD001867.

28. R. F. Anton et al., "Combined pharmacotherapies and behavioral interventions for alcohol dependence: The COMBINE study: A randomized controlled trial." *JAMA* 295, no. 17 (2006): 2003–17.

29. It took until 2012 before release of endorphins in the brain in response to alcohol intake was directly shown in a PET study: J. M. Mitchell et al., "Alcohol consumption induces endogenous opioid release in the human orbitofrontal cortex and nucleus accumbens." *Science Translational Medicine* 4, no. 116 (2012): 116ra6.

30. C. Bond et al., "Single-nucleotide polymorphism in the human mu opioid receptor gene alters beta-endorphin binding and activity: Possible implications for opiate addiction." *Proceedings of the National Academy of Sciences USA* 95, no. 16 (1998): 9608–13.

31. D. W. Oslin et al., "A functional polymorphism of the mu-opioid receptor gene is associated with naltrexone response in alcohol-dependent patients." *Neuropsychopharmacology* 28, no. 8 (2003): 1546–52.

32. C. S. Barr et al., "Association of a functional polymorphism in the mu-opioid receptor gene with alcohol response and consumption in male rhesus macaques." *Archives of General Psychiatry* 64, no. 3 (2007): 369–76.

33. Remember, we all carry two copies of most genes. The exceptions are the few genes that are located on the sex chromosomes, X and Y. The gene for the mu-opioid receptor is not one of those; in humans it is located on chromosome 6.

34. N. B. Urban et al., "Sex differences in striatal dopamine release in young adults after oral alcohol challenge: A positron emission tomography imaging study with [11C] raclopride." *Biological Psychiatry* 68, no. 8 (2010): 689–96. It has been suggested that this difference may contribute to the 2:1 ratio in alcoholism rates between men and women.

35. V. A. Ramchandani et al., "A genetic determinant of the striatal dopamine response to alcohol in men." *Molecular Psychiatry* 16, no. 8 (2011): 809–17.

36. A. J. Chamorro et al., "Association of mu-opioid receptor (OPRM1) gene polymorphism with response to naltrexone in alcohol dependence: A systematic review and meta-analysis." *Addiction Biology* 17, no. 3 (2012): 505–12.

37. A. B. Whitworth et al., "Comparison of acamprosate and placebo in long-term treatment of alcohol dependence." *Lancet* 347, no. 9013 (1996): 1438–42; H. Sass et al., "Relapse prevention by acamprosate: Results from a placebo-controlled study on alcohol dependence." *Archives of General Psychiatry* 53, no. 8 (1996): 673–80.

38. B. J. Mason and P. Lehert, "Acamprosate for alcohol dependence: A sex-specific meta-analysis based on individual patient data." *Alcoholism: Clinical and Experimental Research* 36, no. 3 (2012): 497–508.

39. B. J. Mason et al., "Effect of oral acamprosate on abstinence in patients with alcohol dependence in a double-blind, placebo-controlled trial: The role of patient motivation." *Journal of Psychiatric Research* 40, no. 5 (2006): 383–93.

40. R. F. Anton et al., "Combined pharmacotherapies and behavioral interventions for alcohol dependence: The COMBINE study: A randomized controlled trial." *JAMA* 295, no. 17 (2006): 2003–17.

41. Rats don't have the different genetic variants that in humans determine who will respond to naltrexone.

42. R. Rimondini et al., "Long-lasting increase in voluntary ethanol consumption and transcriptional regulation in the rat brain after intermittent exposure to alcohol." *FASEB Journal* 16, no. 1 (2002): 27–35.

43. R. Spanagel et al., "The clock gene Per2 influences the glutamatergic system and modulates alcohol consumption." *Nature Medicine* 11, no. 1 (2005): 35–42; J. C. Umhau et al., "Effect of acamprosate on magnetic resonance spectroscopy measures of central glutamate in detoxified alcohol-dependent individuals: A randomized controlled experimental medicine study." *Archives of General Psychiatry* 67, no. 10 (2010): 1069–77.

44. B. A. Johnson et al., "Oral topiramate for treatment of alcohol dependence: A randomised controlled trial." *Lancet* 361, no. 9370 (2003): 1677–85; B. A. Johnson et al., "Topiramate for treating alcohol dependence: A randomized controlled trial." *JAMA* 298, no. 14 (2007): 1641–51.

45. G. Addolorato et al., "Effectiveness and safety of baclofen for maintenance of alcohol abstinence in alcohol-dependent patients with liver cirrhosis: Randomised, double-blind controlled study." *Lancet* 370, no. 9603 (2007): 1915–22.

18. PRAY IF YOU WISH, BUT PLEASE TAKE YOUR MEDS FIRST

1. German: "Die Religion . . . ist das Opium des Volkes." Full citation: "Religion is the sigh of the oppressed creature, the heart of a heartless world, and the soul of soulless conditions. It is the opium of the people." Karl Marx, *Deutsch-Französische Jahrbücher* (1844).

2. The actual title of the book is *Alcoholics Anonymous: The Story of How Many Thousands of Men and Women Have Recovered from Alcoholism.*

3. Long-term follow-up studies by, for example, Linda Sobell have shown that this is not quite true. A minority of people with a formal alcoholism diagnosis are in fact able to return to controlled social drinking. These results provoked considerable controversy but have been confirmed by independent studies such as one by Berglund and colleagues in Scandinavia. The problem is, of course, that we have no way of knowing who will be in the minority that will succeed. If it were my life, I would not gamble with that kind of odds.

4. People almost never show this when they publish results of medication studies. One of the few cases where this *was* shown was the groundbreaking paper that evaluated Vivitrol, a depot formulation of naltrexone for alcoholism: J. C. Garbutt et al., "Efficacy and tolerability of long-acting injectable naltrexone for alcohol dependence: A randomized controlled trial." *JAMA* 293, no. 13 (2005): 1617–25.

5. M. Ferri et al., "Alcoholics Anonymous and other 12-step programmes for alcohol dependence." *Cochrane Database of Systematic Reviews* 2006, no. 3: CD005032.

6. As earlier chapters have discussed, methadone and buprenorphine maintenance for opioid addiction are special cases and are highly effective compared to most treatments in clinical medicine.

7. The *AA Grapevine*, at http://www.aagrapevine.org/content/about-us.

8. An area that remains contentious is the use of medications such as methadone and buprenorphine, with their own addictive potential. But even there some interesting developments are under way. I will return to those shortly.

9. At the time of this writing, the study is still ongoing.

10. If I understand things correctly, the original idea was to make the Old Lodge a retreat for clergy with alcoholism. This was soon broadened to include other professionals.

11. Although contracts with insurers are good in the sense that they expand access to treatment, they are not without their complications. The negotiated contract reimbursement is heavily discounted, increasing the pressure for cost savings or greater revenue elsewhere.

INDEX

bloodletting, 190
Bloom, Floyd, 81, 83
body state, 95
body sway, 153
Bohman, Michael, 142–45, 147
Bosch, Hieronymus, 190
b-processes, 83
Bradley, Nelson, 244
brain: changes in as triggered by addic-
    tion, 257–58; chemical anatomy of,
    61–62; healthy one as compared to
    addicted one, 83; as master gland,
    128; plasticity of, 258. *See also specific*
    components of the brain
brain imaging, 116–19, 133, 160, 246
brain mechanisms (of addiction), 51
brain microdialysis, 64
brain reward systems/circuitry, 51, 58–74,
    82, 85, 98, 118, 153, 183, 207
brief intervention, 195–96
British, and opium trade, 166
Buddhism, 57, 204
built-in brake (on alcohol intake), 153
buprenorphine, 9, 171, 186, 210–12, 213–15,
    252, 257, 261
butanol, 179
Butler, Pat, 252
Butler Center for Research, 245

Campral (acamprosate), 224
cannabinoids, 30
cannabis, 9, 19, 229
Cannabis indica, 19
Cannabis sativa, 19
Carlos (vignette), 89–92, 96, 103
Carlsson, Arvid, 61
Caron, Marc, 176
Catholic Church, 165
Centers for Disease Control and Pre-
    vention (CDC), 4, 5
cerebral cortex, 119, 133
CET. *See* cue exposure therapy

Champix (varenicline), 216
change, readiness for, 192
Chantix (varenicline), 216
charlatans (in treatment field), 262–63
Chinese, opium use, 166
choices: addicts as often making bad
    ones, 92–93; facing investigators
    studying new alcoholism treatment,
    110
Christianity, on happiness, 58
clinical alcoholism, 29
clinical diagnostic criteria, 20, 22–23
Cloninger, Robert, 144
coca, 171–74
Coca-Cola, 174
cocaine: alcohol as greater cause of
    death/disability, 9; barriers to obtain-
    ing/using as higher than for nicotine,
    20; as binding to more than one place
    in the brain, 176; in Coca-Cola, 174;
    deaths from as compared to deaths
    from prescription opioid analgesics,
    214; different methods of using, 175;
    effect of on mesolimbic dopamine
    transmission, 65; euphoria experience
    from, 20; experiments on monkeys
    with, 73; extraction of, 174; harm to
    self and others inflicted by as less
    than that of alcohol, 16; as having
    unusual chemistry, 175; high produced
    as more uniform than that from
    heroin or morphine, 177; medications
    for addiction to, 229; minority of users
    as developing particularly destructive
    relationship with, 20; naming of, 174;
    number of users of, 178; as out-
    lawed most places outside of South
    America, 174; in Pemberton's French
    Wine Coca, 174; as producing anxiety
    and low mood, 80; as the prototypical
    psychostimulant, 179; as psychostimu-
    lant, 164; as reliably producing a high,

Edwards, Griffith, 18, 21, 29, 30
EEA. *See* equal environment assumption
EEG. *See* electroencephalogram
effectiveness, compared to efficacy, 280n2
effects: alcohol, multifaceted effects
    of, 183; dampening effects, 183, 184;
    drug effects, as interaction between
    molecules and brains they hit,
    168; mind-altering drug effects,
    19; motor-stimulating effects, 183,
    184; pleasurable effects, 67, 83, 168;
    psychotropic drug effects, 19, 85, 165;
    sleep-inducing effects, 184
ego weakness, 78
Egypt, distilled spirits, 180
Eisenberger, Naomi, 132
electroencephalogram (EEG), 46
Eli Lilly, 246
emotions, theory of, 197
empathy, importance of provider's
    expression of, 194
endocrinology, 35, 129
endogenous opioids, 69, 165, 220, 222
endophenotypes, 155
endorphin receptors, 207
endorphins, 68, 69, 73, 183, 207
end-stage diseases, 29
environmental component/factors/influ-
    ences/variables, 19, 37, 140, 141, 145,
    146, 148
enzymes, 157, 159, 264
Epstein, David, 201
equal environment assumption (EEA),
    277n8
Eric (vignette), 12–15, 24, 27, 28
Erickson, Carlton, 247
Erythroxylon coca, 171
escalation, 25, 68, 73, 226
ethyl alcohol (ethanol), 179
euphoria, 20, 82, 168, 169, 172
European Medicines Agency, 110
Evans, Chris, 70

evidence-based medicine, 186, 188–89,
    197, 199, 204, 208, 237, 238, 240, 245,
    249
excited, becoming, 182
executive functions, 96
exons, 156, 157
extended residential care, 14
externalizing psychiatric disorders, 151,
    152
extinction (of behavior), 108, 109, 120, 121,
    122, 127
extinction–reinstatement model, 115–16
Extracting the Stone of Madness (Bosch),
    190
extrahypothalamic brain regions, 129, 130

facial flushing, 159, 218
Falck, Bengt, 270n10
family history, 162
FDA. *See* U.S. Food and Drug Adminis-
    tration (FDA)
fear learning, 121–22
fears, 53
feelings, ability of medical professionals
    to tune in to those of patients, 42,
    46, 48
fentanyl, 165, 167
fermentation, 180
financial interests, 264
fishbowl reinforcement, 203
fluoresce, 62
flushing reaction, 159, 218
fMRI. *See* functional magnetic reso-
    nance imaging
Ford, Susan, 8, 249
formaldehyde fluorescence method,
    270n10
free base, 175
free will, 41, 43, 44, 47, 48, 103, 193
Frigo, Dan, 252
frontal lobes, 94, 95, 97, 99, 102, 109, 117,
    118, 122, 133, 183

therapies (*continued*)
   talk therapy, 13; third-wave cognitive-
   behavioral therapies, 204; voucher-
   based reinforcement therapy, 203
third-wave cognitive-behavioral therapies, 204
Thompson, Hazel, 250
Thorndyke, Edward Lee, 58
Thorsell, Annika, 222, 223
thyroid gland, 128
thyrotropin releasing factor (TRF), 128
thyrotropin releasing hormone (TRH),
   128
tolerance, 170, 171, 199
topiramate, 228
transcranial magnetic stimulation
   (TMS), 119
transmitters, 51, 157, 177, 182. *See also*
   neurotransmitters
treatment: access to as lacking, 28;
   antihypertensive treatment, 27, 30;
   behavioral treatments, 119–10, 186,
   188, 205; challenges facing studies
   of, 186–87; costs of, 188, 261; costs of
   research studies on, 228–29; diffi-
   culty in getting funding for, 253; for
   hypertension as example of potential
   for addiction, 39–40; importance of
   building an alliance in, 45; importance of long-term disease management approaches, 198; importance of
   patient taking responsibility in, 45;
   importance of relationship building
   in, 191–94; importance of working together in, 45; as an industry,
   9; key elements of effective ones,
   197; medical treatments seen as not
   appropriate or effective, 39; megabuck industry based on provision
   of, 189; Minnesota Model, 244, 245,
   252, 253; most commonly offered
   ones, 188; multiphasic approach to,

244; as needing to be tailored to
individual, 191, 226; as needing to
focus on continuing care and disease
management, 40; office-based treatment, 211; outpatient-based treatments, 261; psychosocial treatment,
208–10; recruitment for studies of,
226; resources as scarce for, 9; roles
of various professionals in, 21; studies
evaluating efficacy of, 186; systematic,
structured approaches as ones that
work best, 191
treatment-seeking alcoholics, 29
tremors, 178, 198
trepanation, 190
TRF. *See* thyrotropin releasing factor
TRH. *See* thyrotropin releasing hormone
twelve-step facilitation, 232
twelve-step programs/model, 235, 238,
   245, 247, 252
twelve steps of AA, 234–35, 240, 244
twin studies, 145–48, 150

UCLA, 81
Ungerstedt, Urban, 64
University of Pennsylvania Treatment
   Research Center, 36, 110, 114, 221, 248
U.S. Court of Appeals for the Second
   Circuit, ruling on atheist drunk
   driver's constitutional rights, 242
U.S. Food and Drug Administration
   (FDA), 8, 110, 211, 216, 218, 223–24,
   227, 237
U.S. Second Continental Congress, 57
U.S. Supreme Court, on sentencing
   juveniles, 97

Vale, Wylie, 129
Valium, 279n15
varenicline, 186, 216
ventral striatum, 98
ventral tegmental area, 62, 65, 70, 183